RESPIRATORY PHYSIOTHERAPY POCKETBOOK

An On-Call Survival Guide

RESPIRATORY PHYSIOTHERAPY POCKETBOOK

An On-Call Survival Guide

Edited by

Jane Cross EdD, MSc, Grad Dip Phys, MCSP
Senior Lecturer in Physiotherapy,
University of East Anglia, Norwich, UK

Mary-Ann Broad MSc (Critical care), BSc (Physiotherapy), MCSP
Specialist Respiratory Physiotherapist, Queen Elizabeth Hospital,
King's Lynn NHS Trust, King's Lynn, UK;
Associate Tutor in Physiotherapy, University of East Anglia, Norwich, UK

Matthew Quint MCSP, Grad Dip Phys, MPhil
Respiratory Clinical Specialist,
Portsmouth Hospitals NHS trust, Portsmouth, UK

Paul Ritson MCSP, Grad Dip Phys
Clinical Specialist Physiotherapist in Paediatric Intensive Care, Alder Hey
Children's NHS Foundation Trust, Liverpool, UK

Sandy Thomas M Ed MCSP
Associate Lecturer in Physiotherapy,
University of the West of England, Bristol UK

ELSEVIER   Edinburgh   London   New York   Oxford   Philadelphia   St Louis   Sydney   2020

First edition 2004
Second edition 2009
Third edition 2020

Notices

ISBN: 978-0-7020-5507-2

Content Strategist: Poppy Garraway
Content Development Specialist: Veronika Watkins
Content Coordinator: Susan Jansons
Project Manager: Andrew Riley
Design: Patrick Ferguson

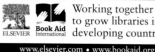

Working together
to grow libraries in
developing countries

www.elsevier.com • www.bookaid.org

Printed in India

Last digit is the print number: 9 8 7 6 5 4 3

CONTENTS

Jayne Anderson PhD, Grad. Dip. Phys.
Lecturer Practitioner Physiotherapist
Physiotherapy Department
Hull Royal Infirmary, Hull, East Yorkshire, UK

Helen Ashcroft-Kelso BSc(hons)
Physiotherapy; MSc Respiratory Practice
Advanced Practice Physiotherapist for Home NIV
Sleep and Ventilation Department
Aintree Hospital NHS Trust, Liverpool, UK

Valerie Ball MSc.
Lecturer in Physiotherapy (retired)
School of Health and Rehabilitation
Keele University, Keele, Staffordshire, UK

Amy Bendall BSc (Hons) Physiotherapy,
MSc Physiotherapy, PgCUTL, FHEA, MCSP
Physiotherapy Lecturer
School of Healthcare Sciences
Cardiff University, Cardiff, UK

Mary-Ann Broad MSc (Critical care), BSc
(Physiotherapy), MCSP
Specialist Respiratory Physiotherapist, Queen
Elizabeth Hospital, King's Lynn NHS Trust, King's
Lynn, UK; Associate Tutor in Physiotherapy,
University of East Anglia, Norwich, UK

Susan Calvert Physiotherapy BSc,
Advanced Physiotherapy MSc
Team Lead Physiotherapist Critical Care
Physiotherapy
Queen Alexandra Hospital, Portsmouth, UK

Vanessa Compton Grad Dip phys
Clinical Specialist Physiotherpist in Critical Care
Physiotherapy
Alder Hey Children's NHS Foundation Trust,
Liverpool, UK

Jane Cross EdD, MSc, Grad Dip Phys,
MCSP
Senior Lecturer in Physiotherapy, University of
East Anglia, Norwich, UK

Alison Draper MCSP, Cert.HE, MSc
Lecturer
Directorate of Physiotherapy
University of Liverpool, Liverpool, UK

Stephen Harden MA (Cantab), MB
BS(Lond), FRCS (Eng), FRCR (UK)
Consultant Cardiothoracic Radiologist
Wessex Cardiothoracic Centre,
Southampton, UK

Claire Hepworth Bsc (hons) Physiotherapy
PHYSIOTHERAPY
Alder Hey Hospital, Liverpool, UK

Kate Jones Bsc
Physiotherapist
Physiotherapy
Cardiff and Vale UHB, Cardiff, UK

Joules Lodge BSc(Hons) Physiotherapy
Physiotherapy Department
The Queen Elizabeth Hospital, King's Lynn NHS
Trust, King's Lynn, UK

Katharine Malhotra BSc Hons; MSc
Darzi Fellow and Physiotherapist
Therapies
Royal Marsden NHS Foundation Trust,
London, UK

Leanne McCarthy BSc (Hons)
Physiotherapy
Clinical Lead Physiotherapist
Physiotherapy Department
Blackpool Teaching Hospitals, Blackpool, UK

Ellie Melkuhn Bsc (Hons) Physiotherapy
Team Lead Paediatric Respiratory Physiotherapist
Paediatric Physiotherapy
Evelina London Children's Hospital, London, UK

Liz Newton MCSP Grad Dip Phys MSc
Highly specialist physio (medicine NIV) at Bradford
Royal Infirmary

Matthew Quint MCSP, Grad Dip Phys, MPhil
Respiratory Clinical Specialist, Portsmouth
Hospitals NHS trust, Portsmouth, UK

Paul Ritson MCSP, Grad Dip Phys
Clinical Specialist Physiotherapist in Paediatric
Intensive Care, Alder Hey Children's NHS
Foundation Trust, Liverpool, UK

Jennifer Robson BSc (Hons)
Physiotherapy
Respiratory Specialist Physiotherapist
Respiratory Medicine
Portsmouth Hospital NHS Trust, Portsmouth, UK

Sandy Thomas M Ed MCSP
Associate Lecturer in Physiotherapy, University of
the West of England, Bristol UK

Jessica Whibley BSc MCSP
Critical care psychotherapist
The royal marsden NHS trust

The first edition of this book was published back in 2004, as part of a national on-call project within the physiotherapy profession. It aimed to support physiotherapists to safely maintain their respiratory skills, once specialist in other settings, to continue to safely support hospital on call rotas. The maintenance of this broad scope of practice is still considered important to maintain capacity and capability within the profession. The rounded skills set of the physiotherapist have always been the unique selling point of the physiotherapist within healthcare. Now, as the book is published in its third edition and following the first wave of a global pandemic, never has its purpose been more relevant. The book has continued to show its unswerving value to physiotherapists redeployed from across the sectors into intensive care units and acute respiratory units across the world.

We have heard from students, specialists and returners to the profession, how vital this book has been to support their learning, practice and confidence. We now hear the same reports from redeployed staff and returners to the HCPC register, as the first wave of the COVID-19 pandemic slows.

It is good to see this new edition with new chapters showing the evolution of the book from the first edition written 16 years ago and it's continuing, compelling relevance today.

It is a delight to see the editors build on the collaborative approach to the work and the addition of new material to embrace topics such as community respiratory care. The evidence-based content is written by experts across the UK ensuring the content remains up to date and accessible to all. Dr Jane Cross and the team are to be congratulated on this new edition, for enabling me to retire as lead editor, and affording me the honour to now write the foreword.

Beverley Harden MSc, BSc (Hons), FCSP
Allied Health Professions Lead, Health Education England;
Deputy Chief Allied Health Professions Officer, England;
Visiting Professor,
University of Winchester, Winchester, UK

CHAPTER 1

AN INTRODUCTION TO RESPIRATORY CARE

Mary Ann Broad and Jane L. Cross

INTRODUCTION

Many physiotherapists feel daunted at the thought of acute respiratory care and, in particular, being on call. They often feel uncertain that they possess the skills and attributes to care for this patient group (Roskel et al., 2003, Reeve et al., 2012, Bendall et al., 2015). This book aims to provide both students and physiotherapists who are new to, or have little practical experience of respiratory care, a simple and easy to use text to facilitate their assessment and treatment of patients with respiratory problems. It has been written by experienced clinicians and academics, with all chapters peer reviewed. We are particularly indebted to John who, with his extensive experience of respiratory physiotherapy in many settings over several years, provides us with his insights into the patient experience at the end of this chapter.

Previous editions of this text have focussed on being on-call; however, with more hospitals now providing 7-day services and a move towards more community care, it is recognised that patients may be seen anywhere. This book considers acute respiratory care in its many settings as a 24/7, 365-day service and has a new chapter dedicated to the management of patients in the community. Each of the chapters considers patients in different settings and are in a standard format to assist readers to identify key elements of care for these patients.

TRANSFERABLE SKILLS FOR RESPIRATORY CARE

We all have skills that are transferrable across multiple settings and these include:
- infection control
- gaining consent

- clinical reasoning
- communication
- writing accurate documentation

Infection Control

It is easy to forget infection control, but, it is there to protect both you and your patients! Read your organisation's infection control policy. Remember policies vary between organisations and over time. Take precautions to limit the spread of infection in any setting (e.g., effective handwashing, use of masks, goggles or protective clothing and protective gloves, where appropriate).

Sick patients have a reduced capacity to overcome further infection and have numerous access points into which infection can be introduced, including wounds, lines and catheters. Exercise universal precautions for all patients and check for specific instructions if you are called to a patient being nursed in isolation.

Importantly, physiotherapy techniques can increase the quantity of respiratory pathogens exhaled into room air. Patients that are coughing, huffing and expectorating will be sharing their 'bugs'. Ensure you know what specific precautions are expected in addition to universal precautions and where you can access protective equipment as required (e.g., specialist face masks).

Remember!

If you are unsure which precautions to use, ask before commencing your assessment.

Be aware of your own vaccination record and how additional health factors (e.g., your own early pregnancy) might influence your own assessment of risk.

Consent

It is a legal requirement that patients (or parents/guardians in the case of children) must give their consent before you commence any procedure. There is a duty to provide appropriate information so that consent is informed (i.e., the patient or parent/guardian must be aware of the implications of treatment and any possible side effects). Consent may be written, verbal or nonverbal and should be documented in the patient's treatment record. Be aware of your own organisation's policy on consent.

Mentally competent adult patients are entitled to refuse treatment, even when it would clearly benefit their health. The only exception is where the treatment is being provided under mental health legislation.

Patients without capacity/unable to consent
Some adult patients may lack mental capacity to make specific decisions at the time they need to be made. In these circumstances, these adults will not be able to provide valid informed consent or might withhold consent to the proposed treatment. Seek guidance from senior multidisciplinary team (MDT) colleagues if this is a new situation for you. You are not expected to (nor should try to) resolve complex issues of consent on your own.

The Mental Capacity Act 2005, covering Wales and England, provides the legal framework for acting and making decisions on behalf of individuals aged 16 years and over who lack the mental capacity to make particular decisions for themselves. The Adults with Incapacity (Scotland) Act 2000 provides a similar framework for Scotland.

Clinical Reasoning

Acute respiratory care is not just about being able to perform assessment techniques (see Chapter 2 and 3). Asking yourself "what do I do with all this information?" can help you with your clinical reasoning. The implications of the results of your assessment must be considered, linking these to other findings, patient history and the overall clinical picture (context).

At the end of your assessment you should ask yourself:
- What are the patients' problems?
- Are they likely to respond to physiotherapy?
- What precautions should I follow if I intervene?
- What are the techniques I can implement?
- How will I know I was effective with my management?

Problems related to respiratory care are frequently classified as one or more of:
- Sputum retention
- Volume loss
- Increased work of breathing (breathlessness)
- Respiratory failure

These problems are discussed in Chapters 5 to 8. The patient's problems may be complicated by other factors, such as pain, anxiety, other comorbidities, reduced exercise tolerance, weak respiratory or peripheral muscles, functional and mobility limitations or social problems. Once your problem list has been identified, the clinical reasoning process moves on to plan treatment and implementation strategies—the chapters on working in the different settings and case studies can help you with this (see Chapters 9 to 19).

Remember!

You are likely to have many more transferrable skills from other areas of practice than you think! Your patient must be involved in this process and, if they have a chronic respiratory problem, may give you some valuable tips!

Aims of Respiratory Assessment

- Patient safety—to identify patients requiring immediate resuscitation (cardiopulmonary resuscitation)
- To identify the need for respiratory support—such as oxygen therapy or mechanical ventilation
- To identify patients requiring specific physiotherapy treatment for sputum retention, loss of volume or increased work of breathing
- To select appropriate physiotherapy management options for managing sputum retention, loss of volume or increased work of breathing
- To identify patients who need to be referred to the medical team for review, such as patients who do not appear to be on optimum medication (e.g., analgesia or bronchodilators) or those who require further investigations (e.g., deterioration or change in early warning score).
- To determine whether the patient can be safely managed at home, or whether they need to be in hospital (discharge planning for those in hospital, or admission decisions for patients at home)
- To identify any support (e.g., social or medical) the patient may require to be discharged, or remain at home
- To identify and rate the patient's functional ability and level of independence in activities of daily living
- To identify the patient's goals, for example in relation to improving mobility, function or social participation
- To select appropriate physiotherapy management options for enabling functional ability and independence, and make referrals to other MDT members
- To facilitate the prescription of an exercise programme appropriate for the patient's physical, psychologic and social situation

- To assess a patient's suitability for pulmonary rehabilitation
- To choose an outcome measure to use before and after intervention for clinical reasoning, audit or research purposes

Communication
Communication with the multidisciplinary team

A variety of handover and feedback systems are in use clinically; they recognise the importance of high-quality communication and accurate handover of information. These allow clinical staff to handover relevant information about their patient in a clear and logical format, particularly if there has been a change in circumstance and immediate action or escalation of care is required (e.g., referral to critical care). The two currently most commonly in use are SBAR and RSVP (NHSI 2018 and Featherstone 2008).

We all have different communication styles, using these structured tools ensures a logical handover of information presented in a consistent format. They are easy to remember, staff can think and prepare what they want to ask before communication, making handovers quicker and more effective. Any of these handover methods are suitable for all areas of physiotherapy, not just acute care.

Each letter in the SBAR and RSVP acronyms are a heading for the handover process.

SBAR = Situation, Background, Assessment and Recommendation and is from the National Health Service (NHS) Institute for Innovation and Improvement (NHS I, 2018).

RSVP = Reason, Story, Vital Signs, Plan is from the Acute Life-threatening Events Recognition and Treatment (ALERT) course (Featherstone et al., 2008).

Consider how the SBAR format is used in this example:

Situation
Identify both yourself, the patient you are calling about and your concern

Example—This is Mary-Ann the physio on the respiratory ward. I am calling about Mrs Smith she has a NEWS2 score of 9. Her oxygen requirements have increased from 2 litres to 60% to maintain oxygen saturations of 93% and her respiratory rate has risen from 14 to 25. Heart rate is 100 beats per minute and blood pressure is 110/55 mmHg

Background

Give the reason for admission, any significant medical history and what has happened since admission in terms of tests diagnosis, allergies, laboratory tests and other diagnostic results

Example – She was admitted with a community acquired pneumonia 2 days ago and has been on intravenous (IV) antibiotics. Her chest x-ray shows a right lower lobe pneumonia. She has been fine up to this point and is normally fit and well

Assessment

Vital signs, clinical impressions and concerns

Example – Mrs Smith has had stable observations since admission, but her oxygen requirements have crept up significantly over the past 4 hours. Her respiratory rate is now increasing. I am concerned that she is deteriorating and may need transfer to critical care.

Recommendation

Explain what you need, make suggestions on what you want to happen

Example—I would like you to come and review her urgently

At this point the person receiving your call should read back a summary

S—Mrs Smith respiratory ward

B—Admitted with community acquired pneumonia, on IV antibiotics previously stable

A—Sudden deterioration, with increased oxygen requirement and raised respiratory rate, sounds like she is not doing as well

R—I will come immediately. In the meantime, can we up her oxygen to maintain saturations over 94% and ask the ward team to do an arterial blood gas test?

It is important that you communicate clearly with the ward team because they can give you valuable information for your assessment and help you if a second pair of hands is required:

- Speak to the nurse responsible for the patient to gain more detail on the patient's history and any changes
- Do you need the nurse to assist you with your assessment or treatment?
- If the patient is unstable, there is a risk of respiratory or cardiac arrest during your treatment. Ascertain the patient's resuscitation status by checking in the nursing or medical notes. If you are still unclear, discuss with nursing staff or doctor. Make sure that this is the most recent decision.

Communication with the Patient/Relatives

- Explain your role to the patient/parents/guardian to reduce anxiety and distress.
- If relatives are present, ask the patient (if possible) whether or not they would like the relatives present during treatment.
- Relatives sometimes express concern about the proposed treatment, despite a full explanation. In this situation, seek guidance from the MDT on the ward or your senior, who may need to clarify the situation with the relatives.

Should Clinicians Disagree?

Professional autonomy allows physiotherapists the freedom to decide not to treat patients in situations where it is assessed that treatment is inappropriate/contraindicated, despite a doctor's request.

- Discuss your concerns with the doctor.
- Ask why the doctor feels that treatment is indicated?
- Could further investigations, such as chest x-ray, be performed to give clarity to the situation?

If you are still unhappy, phone a senior physiotherapist for support and guidance.

When to Seek Help

Remember other members of the MDT and your senior colleagues are there to support you. You must however, recognise your own scope of practice and in certain situations you should seek their support:

- If the patient is deteriorating rapidly.
- Following assessment, you consider the patient is too unstable to tolerate treatment and may require transfer to critical care for further medical management.
- Following assessment, you are unable to identify the problem and are uncertain about appropriate management.
- You are unsure about specific modifications required for a planned treatment (e.g., the patient has recently had a pneumonectomy).
- You have identified the problem but feel that the treatment is outside your scope of practice.

Documentation

All documentation should be completed in a timely manner, ideally as soon as possible after seeing the patient. Ensure all your documentation is clear and legible. Date, time and sign each new entry (you should also add in a contact bleep number if you carry one) on each page. You should include clear goals, which are **S**pecific, **M**easurable, **A**chievable, **R**ealistic and **T**imed and indicate when you will next review the patient. Discuss the issues with your patient/patient's parents/guardian, this will help you both reach a common consensus, about planned treatment of the patient.

PREPARATION FOR ON CALL

The following section suggests how you can prepare and learn from your experiences to guide your continuing professional development in respiratory care, particularly when on call. Senior staff can facilitate your learning needs and have an obligation to provide appropriate support and training, but it is *your* personal responsibility to ensure you are competent. There are areas you can read up on and prepare in advance; others will need the support of senior colleagues. Each department is different, and you will be able to get information pertinent to your hospital from your manager.

Remember—Be Prepared!
On call policy and guidelines

Request a copy of departmental policy. Read this carefully; it will include valuable information on the operational aspects of the service, such as:

On call period, for example, 5 PM to 9 AM. You must be free to respond to a call at any time within that period.

Referral criteria. There should be clear guidelines for staff regarding the clinical needs of patients who should be referred.

Response time. You should be able to respond within a given time. If not, you will need to stay in hospital accommodation. Discuss this with your manager to help you access an on-call room if necessary.

Health and safety issues, for example, parking and accessing the department at night, working alone, the availability of personal alarms, taxis, infection control, etc.

There are likely to be other contractual issues, for example, payment, time in lieu arrangements and organisation of the rota, which will be local to each hospital.

Identification of Learning Needs

There should be an opportunity to formally assess your knowledge and skills with a senior clinician. This will ensure you have a basic level of competence before commencing on-call and will facilitate identification of learning needs and subsequent development plans. You are expected to have learning needs – qualification as a physiotherapist does not mean you are fully competent or feel confident to work on call! It is useful to have done some preparation to identify your own learning needs; examples might include a SWOT analysis and the Association of Chartered Physiotherapists in Respiratory Care self-assessment tool (Thomas et al., 2006). This can help both you and your senior colleagues to support your learning.

Training and Induction

Your hospital should provide you with an on-call induction, which will offer opportunities to experience different clinical specialities. It is often not possible to have a rotation, which includes critical care before joining an on-call or weekend rota, therefore maximise your learning opportunities during your induction. Remember many skills are transferable.

Familiarise yourself with the following:

- Geography of the hospital and wards
- Treatment guidelines/protocols for your hospital
- Contraindications/precautions to treatment
- Clinical work – you can do this by working alongside a mentor:
  - Observe and discuss assessment
  - Discuss clinical reasoning/problem solving
  - Observe the application of treatment modalities and their evaluation/modification if necessary
- Location and assembly of equipment:
  - For example, cough assist, suction catheters, humidification, and how to access it at night
  - Practise under supervision as systems will vary from Trust to Trust
- How to access patient information.

Take this opportunity to ask lots of questions—remember no question is daft and seniors do appreciate that you may be feeling a little nervous about working out of hours.

Alongside your individualised learning in the clinical environment, each department will have ongoing learning opportunities, such as workshops, lectures or buddy systems designed to update staff on key respiratory topics, but you should revise the basics, such as anatomy and physiology.

Shadow/Buddy Opportunities

Some hospitals offer the opportunity to 'shadow' a senior colleague on call, before being on call independently. Use this opportunity to:

- Observe the on-call procedures, for example, contacting the switchboard, travelling, parking, attending the call and discussing the case, recording attendance/documentation, claiming payment, etc.
- As your confidence builds, take the lead with support and guidance from your seniors. Discuss your clinical reasoning, proposed treatment plan or any problems you have encountered. You may now feel confident with their support on the phone.

Appropriate and Inappropriate Calls

In some hospitals a senior medical doctor must call out the on-call physiotherapist. In others, all calls to the critical care unit must be attended—check the local policy for your hospital. Many conditions benefit from physiotherapy, but for some it is unlikely to help. In many cases, the referrer is asking for your professional opinion/assessment, which is an appropriate part of patient care. Table 1.1 summarises some examples of appropriate and inappropriate calls in the on-call setting. These lists are not exhaustive, and every call must be assessed on its own merits.

The telephone conversation should give you a clearer clinical picture. If you feel the request is inappropriate, explain your reasons and discuss them with the person calling. If the situation is unclear despite your best efforts or the referrer does not agree that physiotherapy is not indicated, you should attend and assess the patient to determine the exact clinical need for treatment. Remember, this is an emergency service for patients who would significantly deteriorate without treatment.

Example Telephone Questions

Using the SBAR format, a suggested method to document your phone call, with prompts on handling the call, is summarised on Table 1.2. This can also be used as an aide memoire for a reflection on your call at a later time.

TABLE 1.1 EXAMPLES OF APPROPRIATE AND INAPPROPRIATE CALLS

CONDITIONS WHERE PHYSIOTHERAPY CAN HELP	CONDITIONS WHERE PHYSIOTHERAPY IS UNLIKELY TO HELP
• Recent aspiration • Recent atelectasis/collapse • Retained secretions causing respiratory distress, e.g., pneumonia, bronchiectasis, CF, COPD with infection or secretions following recent extubation • Poor cough associated with infection and unable to clear • Nonencapsulated lung abscess that will respond to postural drainage • Patients that have benefited from intensive respiratory treatment throughout the day	• Pulmonary oedema – unless infected • Pulmonary embolus • Pulmonary fibrosis • ARDS with minimal secretions • Nonacute, nonproductive COPD • Nonproductive consolidated infection, e.g., TB, pneumonia • Empyema, pleural effusion, pneumothorax – perhaps beneficial if chest drain inserted • Encapsulated lung abscess • Acute bronchospasm, e.g., asthma, unless associated with sputum retention • Patients coughing and expectorating unaided

ARDS, Acute respiratory distress syndrome; CF, cystic fibrosis; COPD, chronic obstructive respiratory disease; TB, tuberculosis.

TABLE 1.2 SBAR FORMAT FOR HANDLING AND RECORDING A REQUEST FOR ON-CALL THERAPY

CALL TIME/DATE:	LOCATION:
Situation: • Patients name? • Where is the patient? • Who is calling? • What are they seeking help/advice for?	
Background: • When did the patient come in? • What has happened/current status? • Any past medical history of note? • What are they like normally? • Previous physio? • Current observations? A,B,C, D etc • Any ceilings to treatment/resus status	
Assessment: • What does the caller think may be wrong? • Do they need you to go in or are they calling for advice? • What is your clinical reasoning at this point?	
Recommendation • Can you give the caller any advice before you get there, e.g., change to humidified oxygen, positioning, analgesia? • Let the caller know if you are on your way and what time will you be there	

THE PATIENTS PERSPECTIVE

As physiotherapists, we may feel daunted about respiratory care, but how do our patients feel about being ill and on the receiving end of our care? It is useful to consider patients stories as they can hugely inform our practice and allow us to reflect on how we treat our patients. John (an experienced service user) has written some of his thoughts on his experiences of physiotherapy. These are his own words.

As someone with a complete C5/6 spinal injury, I have no intercostal muscles and consequently much reduced lung expansion. I cannot cough in the conventional way; I tend to brace myself in my wheelchair and use my diaphragm to push—often with little or no effect. When lying flat in bed, I cannot cough at all. I am telling you this because the prospect of a chest infection is one of my biggest fears. I know that a bad chest infection could potentially kill me. For over 30 years, I struggled hugely with chest infections, maybe only one or two a year, but enough to make my wife and I, on more than one occasion consider moving overseas to avoid winter coughs and colds. Nine months ago, we came to see Tom in the respiratory clinic, and he prescribed me a cough assist machine. There is no question that machine has changed my life. It does not prevent me from getting chest infections, however knowing that it will help clear my chest if and when I get an infection, I am no longer fearful in the way I was previously. It also negates the need for chest physio, thereby eliminating bruised ribs and the guilt of having to wake my wife maybe a dozen times a night to give me chest physio, often with no relief.

You worry about cross-contamination, with bugs being transmitted from the patient, but that works both ways. So, almost on a daily basis, I 'assess' the people I come into contact with and, as I have got older and less afraid to speak my mind, it has been known that I decline a meeting or an examination by someone who is exhibiting cold or flu symptoms. Even to the point where I will wear a face mask in the house if my wife or my son get colds. My immune system is greatly reduced by my disability, so I have to be vigilant at all times.

For me personally, coughs and colds go to my chest very quickly. The usual cycle from feeling a sore throat to getting a chest infection is about a week. Once I get a chest infection, they last approximately 3 weeks. Interestingly, when I say chest infection, mine are often viral and not treatable with antibiotics. Only if they get worse, do antibiotics have any effect.

As a patient, the sensation I get with a chest infection is one of panic, drowning, inability to sleep and tiredness and fatigue as my body tries and fails, to cough. Assisted physio is one option but I must stress it can be painful, incredibly tiring and futile on many occasions. Chest physio may ultimately help loosen sticky mucus in the lung, but it could be an hour before I'm in a position to cough up any mucus. And it can be demoralising too because, the moment that mucus is cleared, in a matter of minutes the next bubble starts to tickle and grow in my lung. For me personally, if I require an out-of-hours intervention, the prospect of being visited for 30 minutes or maybe an hour, does little for me. Because in reality I really do need someone with me or at least nearby, for the duration of the illness.

References

Bendall, A.L., Watt, A., 2015. Final year physiotherapy undergraduate students' perceptions of preparedness for emergency on-call respiratory physiotherapy: a questionnaire survey. J. Assoc. Chartered. Physiotherap. Respir. Care. 48, 4–13.

Featherstone, P., Chalmers, T., Smith, G.B., 2008. RSVP: a system for communication of deterioration in hospital patients. Br. J. Nurs. 17 (13), 860–864.

NHS Improvement, 2018. SBAR Communication Tool- Situation, Background, Assessment, Recommendation. https://improvement.nhs.uk/resources/sbar-communication-tool/.

Reeve, J., Skinner, M., Lee, A., Wilson, L., Alison, J.A., 2012. Investigating factors influencing 4th-year physiotherapy students' opinions of cardiorespiratory physiotherapy as a career path. Physiotherap. Theory. Pract. 28 (5), 391–401.

Roskell, C., Cross, V., 2003. "Student perceptions of cardio-respiratory physiotherapy" Physiotherapy 89 (1), 2–12.

Thomas, S., Broad, M.A., Cross, J., Harden, B., Quint, M., Ritson, P., 2006. Acute respiratory/on call physiotherapy – self-evaluation of competence questionnaire. Available online www.acprc.org.uk/dmdocuments/competence_questionnaire.pdf.

RESPIRATORY ASSESSMENT

Matthew J. Quint and Sandy Thomas

The goal of assessment is to establish the clinical situation, the indications and contraindications to treatment. This starts from the moment the referral is received. Not all information is required for all patients, so tailor your assessment to the patient.

There are two main approaches to acute care assessment; you should follow local guidelines on which assessment format to use:

1. The ABCDE assessment process—used initially to determine whether the patient is in immediate danger, however, many hospitals also use this approach to organise their full assessment (see Chapter 13, Critical care).

2. A systems-based approach, outlined in this chapter, facilitates a structured, comprehensive and systematic approach, which some physiotherapists prefer.

In any clinical situation, a 'quick check' from the end of the bed is crucial to establish the stability of the patient and indicate how quickly you should act and how ill the patient is. Although your focus is physiotherapy problems and treatment strategies, your first priority is to ensure patient safety. Your first question should be: 'Is the patient in immediate danger?'

Patient A

- It is 20.00 hours and you are called to see an 84-year-old male on a medical ward. He was admitted yesterday with community-acquired pneumonia, and was treated earlier in the day by the ward physiotherapist. The nurse in charge reports he has dropped his oxygen saturation and sounds bubbly. She has asked that you review this patient.
- He has a previous stroke and mild dementia. Although he is for full and active treatment, he is not considered appropriate for resuscitation
- On arrival at the ward, the registrar is reviewing the notes, and the nursing staff are handing over to the night staff.
  What should you do now?

ABCDE assessment process:

A—Airway, is it patent and protected?

If not: Call for help and establish an airway.

B—Breathing, are they ventilating effectively? What are their oxygen saturations and are they on oxygen?

If not: Call for help and support ventilation.

C—Circulation, do they have an adequate cardiac output?

If not: Call for help and support output.

If the answer to any of these questions is 'no', something immediately needs to be done to stabilise the patient.

Could you recognise these signs, and would you know how to address them? If not, you need to update your basic life support. Refer to the ABCDE approach (Resuscitation council UK)[1], and to the respiratory and circulatory sections in this chapter.

For Patient A, start with ABC, then perform a full systems-based assessment.

Patient A has audible crackles at the mouth, is using his accessory muscles and breathing very shallowly. It is clear his airway is compromised and needs to be cleared immediately to ensure his safety before the assessment can proceed.

If you are unsure, do not be afraid to call for help.

Remember you do not have sole responsibility for the care of the patient. Other members of the team are there to support you and you are there to support them.

Once you have established that the patient is in no immediate danger you should continue with:

D—Disability, assess their conscious level; and
E—Exposure, look at the whole patient.

A Systems based assessment:

Be systematic in your approach; include each physiologic system, cardiovascular, renal and so on.

SUBJECTIVE HISTORY

Consider: What has changed? Why has it changed? How is this impacting on the patient and/or the clinical intervention?

HISTORY OF PRESENT CONDITION

Reflect whether the patient's current situation may relate to any of the four key respiratory physiotherapy problems. You can also determine whether the patient is deteriorating, stable or improving.

Focus on key respiratory symptoms:

Wheeze

What is the cause (swelling, bronchospasm or sputum)?
What is most likely in your patient (are there clues in the past medical history)?

Shortness of Breath

If shortness of breath at rest (or minimal exertion) is not normal for the patient, this is cause for concern and could lead to fatigue if not addressed.

What can you do to relieve the work of breathing?

Cough

A cough is a normal important part of airway clearance, it can be a reflex or voluntary and will only clear central airways.

Is it effective? Productive or dry? Is the patient wasting energy with an unproductive cough and getting fatigued?

Sputum

How much is coughed up each day, what colour is it, how viscous, is it difficult to clear? Does the patient have an airway clearance regimen they usually perform and is it working now?

Chest Pain

Cardiac chest pain may be crushing and central, radiating to the left arm and neck, but it can present in other areas including the jaw and between the scapular (if this is new it should be highlighted to the medical team).

For other sources of pain, ensure there is adequate analgesia to allow treatment, consider the site, irritability and nature. How does it change with the respiratory cycle? Can the patient cough effectively?

PAST MEDICAL HISTORY

You need to establish how serious the current episode is and whether you can draw on previous physiotherapy interventions to find the most effective treatment.

Think about:
- Underlying pathologies that may impact on the patient's care?
- Contraindications to treatment?
- Allergies?
- Previous/similar episodes?
- Treatments the patient has had before?
- Physiotherapy treatments the patient has had before? How did they respond?

DRUG HISTORY

This should include oxygen prescription and target saturations.

Often patients will say they are fit and well but report a long list of medications that indicate other pathologies.

Consider if any drugs could facilitate physiotherapy, for example, nebulised saline, additional analgesia.

SOCIAL HISTORY

What is the patient normally like? Is there a history of smoking?

Remember, smoking is the major cause of chronic lung disease.

OBJECTIVE HISTORY

Will identify the current situation. Look for trends over time, is the patient compromised, improving, unchanged or deteriorating?

The two components in this part of the assessment are:
- Observation—including charts
- Physical examination.

Remember it is easy to dive in, but it is important to take a considered approach (Table 2.1).

TABLE 2.1	A CONSIDERED APPROACH TO ASSESSMENT
Stop	Take stock of the situation and what you have discovered so far
Look	Look at the patient and the information available from charts and monitors carefully
Listen	Listen to what the patient tells you and what you hear on auscultation
Feel	Examine them systematically. Remember your hands may tell you more than a stethoscope
Think	Relate your findings to the patient's history What potential problems have you identified and are they consistent with the history? Can you manage this patient? Do you need help?

TABLE 2.2	GENERAL OBSERVATIONS
GENERAL	
Comfort	Does the patient look comfortable, or unwell and distressed, do you need to address this first?
Size	Are they obese? Are there manual handling and/or respiratory implications? Are they malnourished, if so they may fatigue quickly.
Position	What position are they in? This impacts on both lung volume and work of breathing. (See Chapter 6, Management of Volume Loss)
Posture	Do they have a kyphosis or scoliosis? Chest wall deformities are associated with volume loss and respiratory failure. (See Chapter 6 Management of Volume Loss and Chapter 8 Management of Respiratory Failure)
Apparatus	What equipment, drains or lines are attached to them, are they switched on and working properly. If you are unfamiliar with equipment—*ask*.

This approach is used as you work through the body systems (Tables 2.3–2.6).

General observation allows you to take in the overall situation of the patient, including the equipment surrounding them, the personnel and relatives or carers who may be present (see Table 2.2). Issues of consent and treatment should be directed to the patient, but you may need to involve others in these discussions.

CARDIOVASCULAR SYSTEM

This gives you more information about the patient's stability and ability to tolerate physiotherapy.

Remember!

Things may change quickly so keep monitoring for deterioration (see Table 2.3).
- Look for trends
- What is their normal status?
- What physiologic stress is the patient under?
- Is their circulation becoming compromised?

ELECTROCARDIOGRAM MONITORING

You are not responsible for diagnosis. If something does not look right, ask—you may be the first person to have seen a new problem. First check the 'stickies' or electrocardiogram (ECG) dots and leads are attached. Is the trace regular? Is it fast or slow? A serious dysrhythmia in one person may have no adverse effects in another, so look at the patient!

Blood pressure is key when deciding the importance of any dysrhythmia. Consider the patients colour, temperature and conscious level. Trends in the dysrhythmia are also important.
- Has it just occurred?
- Did it occur suddenly or gradually?
- Is it getting more frequent?
- How is your treatment affecting it?

Pay attention to dysrhythmias that have recently appeared or are getting more frequent. Remember, manual chest treatments will affect the ECG trace, so allow the trace to settle before interpreting abnormalities.

NEUROLOGIC SYSTEM

Considered in more detail in Chapter 14.
See Table 2.4 for neurologic observations.

TABLE 2.3 CARDIOVASCULAR OBSERVATIONS

OBSERVATIONS	RELEVANCE
Heart rate (HR) Bradycardia HR <50 beats/min Tachycardia HR >100 beats/min	Consider predicted 'maximum' (220 – age) and how much more you may increase this during physiotherapy?
Blood pressure (BP) Normally 95/60–140/90 mmHg	Increases with age. The significance of abnormal values depends on the patient's normal. Note change or trends
Hypotension <95/60 mmHg (Adults)	A patient whose pulse is higher than their systolic blood pressure (at rest) is significantly compromised. This needs to be addressed quickly by the medical team. Avoid physiotherapy until blood pressure is stable
Hypertension >140/90 mmHg	Significance depends on patient's age and their 'normal' values. A diastolic of >95 mmHg warrants caution
Inotropic drugs	Is the patient on drugs to support their BP? Their cardiovascular system may be less stable, so take care with treatments (Critical Care see Chapter 13)
Central venous pressure (CVP)	Gives an indication of overall fluid filling the circulatory system and is measured invasively using a central line Low values—patient may be dehydrated or have poor venous return High values—may be caused by positive pressure ventilation, fluid overload or heart failure
Capillary refill time	Measured by asking the patient to hold their finger at the level of their heart, you pinch it and hold for 5 seconds. After letting go, count how long it takes for blanching to clear, normally ≤3 seconds. If it takes longer, suggests poor blood flow, which could be related to inadequate circulation overall Feeling the patient's hands/feet will give you an idea how well perfused the patient is—the colder they are, the worse the circulation is
Oedema	Is there any oedema and where is it? Oedema in both legs might suggest heart failure Generalised oedema may affect the lungs, with crackles heard on auscultation sounding similar to sputum retention, but this will not improve with physiotherapy treatment

TABLE 2.3 CARDIOVASCULAR OBSERVATIONS—cont'd

OBSERVATIONS	RELEVANCE
Haematology	If white cell count is increased there may be infection If platelets are low, there may be an increase in risk of bleeding This may contraindicate manual techniques Note the clotting time/international normalised ratio
Temperature	Look for hyper or hypothermia—either could compromise the patient's tolerance of intervention

TABLE 2.4 NEUROLOGIC OBSERVATIONS

OBSERVATIONS	RELEVANCE
ACVPU A quick and easy assessment of a patient's overall neurologic status	**A** = patient is **A**lert **C** = **C**onfused (assume it is new until proven otherwise) **V** = responds to **V**oice **P** = only responds to **P**ain **U** = **U**nresponsive If the patient's status is lower than 'Alert' and the team are not aware, report immediately. Take note if the neurologic status deteriorates during your assessment/treatment and alert the team. Unresponsive patients need their airway protected—consider an oral airway, or the recovery position if appropriate
GCS (Glasgow Coma Scale) A detailed and quick assessment of neurologic status scores between 3–15	Tests best response of: Eyes (Scored 1–4) Verbal (Scored 1–5) Motor (Scored 1–6)
Pupils	Look at size and reactivity For example, pinpoint pupils may suggest too much morphine, unequal pupils may indicate neurologic changes
Neurologic observations Intercranial pressure (ICP) and cerebral perfusion pressure (CPP)	Report any change Use to monitor adverse effects of physiotherapy (Neurology—see Chapter14)

Continued

TABLE 2.4	NEUROLOGIC OBSERVATIONS—cont'd
OBSERVATIONS	RELEVANCE
Drugs/sedation	Is patient receiving any sedative drugs? What is the level of sedation (does your hospital score sedation levels?) Sedation may affect ability to participate in treatment or may be needed if patient is agitated Heavily sedated patients may not be able to cooperate with active treatments (e.g., active cycle of breathing technique)
Drugs—paralysing	Is patient receiving any paralysing agents? Paralysed patients cannot breathe or cough for themselves. Take extra care when removing from ventilator to bag them and when moving them (joint protection, reassurance)
Tone	Changes in tone or patterning indicates severity of neurologic damage and implications for moving the patient. How do they handle?
Blood glucose	Low values impair the patient's neurologic status. May need to be addressed immediately
Pain	Are they in pain? Is a scoring system being used? What analgesia is being used? What dose? What route? Is it enough? Ask for pain control to be increased if necessary

There remains debate regarding the most effective and quick assessment of neurologic status. Some units may choose 'ACVPU' and others the GCS. You should follow local guidelines.

RENAL SYSTEM

Patients with renal failure may require different forms of support. This frequently involves the insertion of a large-bore cannula (e.g., Vas-Cath). Care must be taken while handling these patients to ensure these are not occluded or dislodged. Consider fluid balance and urine output (see Table 2.5).

TABLE 2.5 RENAL OBSERVATIONS

OBSERVATIONS	RELEVANCE
Urine output Normal is 0.5–1.0 mL per kg of body weight per hour	If there is no urine output, this does not necessarily mean the patient is in renal failure Is there a catheter in situ, is it blocked, is it in the right place? Poor output can be related to shock and risk of cardiovascular insufficiency, discuss with team **! Remember**: A change in urine output is a sensitive marker of patient improvement or deterioration
Fluid balance chart Look at cumulative balance, i.e., input vs. output (check totals include all sources of fluid loss)	Overhydration (risks pulmonary oedema and crackles not caused by sputum) Underhydration (risks dehydration and viscous sputum) Check for low albumen levels as protein levels affect fluid distribution. This can mean fluid moves into extravascular spaces, producing circulatory compromise, despite an apparently normal fluid balance

Musculoskeletal

Key questions:

- Is there a history of trauma past or present? Will this impact on your planned treatment?
- Is there a potential spinal fracture? Has the spine been 'cleared'? If unsure treat as unstable (see Chapter 14).
- Injuries can be missed initially so do not be surprised if additional injuries are discovered (e.g., ligamentous disruption) and ensure they are reported.
- Identify any fractures, soft tissue injuries and how they are being managed. External fixators and traction may limit positioning the patient.

RESPIRATORY

The observations on Table 2.6 should guide you towards any key physiotherapy problems.

Airway must be assessed. Is it patent and protected?

TABLE 2.6   RESPIRATORY OBSERVATIONS

OBSERVATIONS	RELEVANCE
Mode of ventilation	Spontaneous, noninvasive or invasive? (NIV—Respiratory Failure, see Chapter 8; Invasive ventilation C-ritical Care, see Chapter 13).
Respiratory rate Adult normal 12–16 breaths per minute	Compare the documented rate to the rate that you measure. Expect increases when demand increases
Increased rate	Check partial pressure of carbon dioxide ($PaCO_2$). If low, are they hyperventilating because of stress? Anxiety? Pain? Fever? Low partial pressure of oxygen (PaO_2) *and* high respiratory rate indicates cardiac or respiratory problem
>30 per min trend increasing *Becoming critical*	Check gases for signs of respiratory failure
Reduced rate *Could be critical*	Oversedation? Neurologic incident? Fatigue? Check gases for signs of respiratory failure
Work of breathing	Use of accessory muscles (including the abdominals during expiration) and pursed lipped breathing may suggest fatigue
Pattern	Irregular breathing pattern may be linked to fatigue or neurologic damage
Expansion	Is it equal? Decreased movement may be linked to loss of volume (see Chapter 6)
Oxygen therapy	Take into account any oxygen patient is receiving when interpreting oxygen saturation Sp/PaO_2. Is current therapy adequate? Hypoxemia is classified as an inability to keep PaO_2 above 8 kPa. (See Respiratory Failure, Chapter 8)

TABLE 2.6   RESPIRATORY OBSERVATIONS—cont'd

OBSERVATIONS	RELEVANCE
Pulse oximetry (SpO_2) normal 95%–98%	Look for trends and report any deterioration (e.g., oxygen saturation [sats] of 90% may be less worrying than sats which have dropped from 98% to 92%) *In acute illness* <92% may be significant but expect lower values in elderly patients and during sleep *Patients with reduced cardiac output* Slight hypoxemia <94% may be significant Patients who are peripherally shut down may not have adequate blood flow to detect saturations accurately, check trace! *Chronic chest patient* Hypoxemia may not be significant until <80%–85%. Compare with 'usual' values for patient (has the team set accepted parameters?)
Arterial blood gases	See interpretation Fig. 2.1
Chest x-ray	Is there any indication of specific problems? Are there changes? See system for interpretation Table 2.7 and (see Chapter 4, Chest X-Rays)
Cough	Is cough effective and patient at risk of sputum retention?
Sputum	Note, viscosity, colour, smell, volume, presence of haemoptysis How easy is it to clear and is there risk of sputum retention?
Chest shape	Chest wall defects will reduce lung volumes and predispose the patient to increased work of breathing
Hands	Peripheral cyanosis, clubbing, temperature, nicotine stains May suggest a chronic problem?

Continued

TABLE 2.6   RESPIRATORY OBSERVATIONS—cont'd

OBSERVATIONS	RELEVANCE
Surgical wounds	Consider site and procedure the patient has undergone (see Chapter 14 and 15) Pain from the wound and the anaesthetic can reduce lung volumes and lead to sputum retention.
Intercostal drains	Are they present, draining, bubbling or swinging? (see Chapter 15). Consider the effects of pain and immobility
Lung function tests	Vary with age, sex and height; compare with predicted normal values Values often found in notes are written as a percentage of predicted for patient's age sex and height. Is this a chronic problem?
Hemoglobin 12–18 g/100 mL	High values suggest polycythaemia Low values suggest anaemia—consider this before interpreting SpO_2. A patient with low saturations may have normal oxygen content available to the tissues if the haemoglobin levels are very high

If there is an artificial airway, what type is it? Endotracheal tube, tracheostomy, nasal or oral airway?

See Chapter 4, Chest X-Rays. A systematic approach to reviewing means you are less likely to miss something (see table 2.7). This a suggested system; if you use another, and are happy using it, continue to do so.

PHYSICAL EXAMINATION

Surface anatomy/surface marking

Good knowledge of normal surface anatomy will help your assessment.

The guidance in Fig. 2.3 is for normal adults. Pathology may change anatomy and you must adapt your assessment as appropriate.

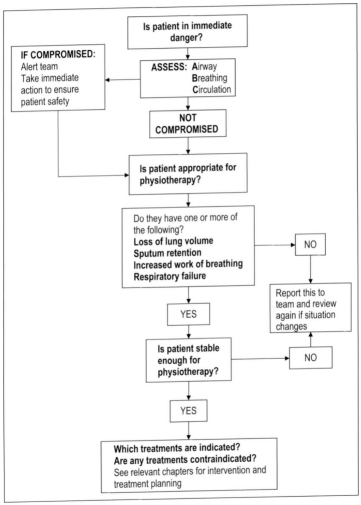

Fig. 2.1 • Decision making process.

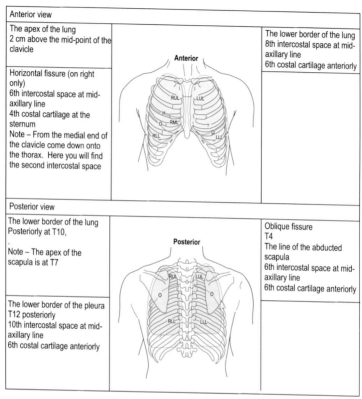

Anterior view		
The apex of the lung 2 cm above the mid-point of the clavicle	**Anterior**	The lower border of the lung 8th intercostal space at mid-axillary line 6th costal cartilage anteriorly
Horizontal fissure (on right only) 6th intercostal space at mid-axillary line 4th costal cartilage at the sternum Note – From the medial end of the clavicle come down onto the thorax. Here you will find the second intercostal space		
Posterior view		
The lower border of the lung Posteriorly at T10, . Note – The apex of the scapula is at T7	**Posterior**	Oblique fissure T4 The line of the abducted scapula 6th intercostal space at mid-axillary line 6th costal cartilage anteriorly
The lower border of the pleura T12 posteriorly 10th intercostal space at mid-axillary line 6th costal cartilage anteriorly		

Fig. 2.2 • Surface marking.

Palpation

Consider the elements in Tables 2.8 and 2.9.

AUSCULTATION

Describe breath sounds and added sounds (Tables 2.10–2.13).

TABLE 2.7 A SYSTEM FOR CHEST X-RAY INTERPRETATION— QUESTIONS TO ASK

KEEPING THE FILM IN CONTEXT	ABOUT THE FILM ITSELF	
Who is the film of?	**A**—**A**lignment and **A** quick look	Is it a straight film? Is there anything obvious that jumps out?
What was the x-ray of?	**B**—**B**ones	Are they all there and intact?
Where was it taken?	**C**—**C**ardiac	Is it in the correct position, the right size and clear borders?
When was it taken?	**D**—**D**iaphragm	Is it in the correct position; are there clear contours and angles?
Why was it taken?	**E**—**E**xpansion and **E**xtrathoracic structures	Is the chest well expanded? Examine structures outside of the thorax
How was it taken?	**F**—lung **F**ields	Are the lung fields clear and do they extend to the edge of the thorax
	G—**G**adgets	Are there any lines, drains, tubes, sutures, clips etc?

TABLE 2.8 PALPATION

Temperature	Does the patient feel hot/cold? Compare central to peripheral
Oedema	Is there obvious central or peripheral oedema? If so, how might this impact on treatment?
Trachea	Is it central? If not, do you feel it has been pushed to one side, for example by a mass or pulled by collapse? Is this new?
Expansion	Is it equal and consistent during inspiratory and expiratory cycle?
Tactile fremitus	Can you feel any crackles under your hands? Use this to guide later aspects of the examination (percussion note and auscultation)

TABLE 2.9   PERCUSSION NOTE

Percussion note	Perform by placing a finger horizontally on the chest wall between two ribs and tapping with sharply with a finger or knuckle of the other hand
Resonant because of air in thorax	Air in lung (normal)
Hyperresonant	Air between the pleura (pneumothorax) Overexpanded lung (Emphysema)
A dull sound because of fluid or solid underlying tissue	This is normal if over liver or abdominal contents Over lungs: pleural effusion or consolidation

TABLE 2.10   BREATH SOUNDS

BREATH SOUNDS	INDICATES
Normal breath sounds Soft, muffled, louder on inspiration, fade in expiration, Ratio of inspiration to expiration = 1:2	Normal turbulence in the large airways
Bronchial breathing Expiration louder and longer with pause between inspiration and expiration, Heard normally over trachea	If heard over lung fields: Consolidation Collapse without a sputum plug May also be heard at the lip of a pleural effusion
Breath sounds quiet or absent? Poor expansion Low lung volumes Atelectasis	May be caused by: • Shallow breathing • Poor positioning • Collapse with complete obstruction of airway • Sounds reduced by hyperinflation • Sounds reduced by pleura, chest wall (obese or muscular patients, pleural effusion, pneumothorax, haemothorax) • Pneumothorax

TABLE 2.11   ADDED SOUNDS—CRACKLES

Crackles	Cause and clinical relevance Short, nonmusical, popping sounds, fine or coarse	
Fine crackles Reopening of airways sounds like rubbing hair next to your ear	• Atelectasis • Intraalveolar oedema • Secretions small airways	• Short, sharp • At lung periphery • Lessen with a deep breath • "Tissue paper" • Do not resolve with deep breath or cough • Late inspiration (Note: this could also be caused by interstitial fibrosis) • High pitched • Periphery • Clear with cough
Coarse crackles Sounds like pouring milk on rice krispies	Obstruction more proximal and larger airways with sputum. May be during inspiration, as well as expiration	• Early expiratory—in central airways • Late expiratory— in more peripheral airways • Large deep sound • Changes/clears with coughing

! REMEMBER: Crackles are only heard if the velocity of air is adequate and breath sounds are audible

TABLE 2.12   ADDED SOUNDS—WHEEZE

Wheezes	Cause and clinical relevance Musical sounds because of vibration of wall of narrowed airway	
High Pitched Wheeze	Bronchospasm	• Potential increased work of breathing
Low pitched wheeze	Sputum	• Disrupted turbulent flow • Change with coughing
Localised wheeze	Tumour or foreign body	• Limited to a local area on auscultation

TABLE 2.13	OTHER SOUNDS	
OTHER SOUNDS	SOUNDS LIKE	CAUSE
Pleural rub	Creaking/rubbing (like walking boots in snow) Localised/generalised Soft/loud Equal inspiration to expiration	Inflammation of pleura Infection Tumour
Stridor	Sound of constant pitch during both inspiration and expiration in upper airways	Croup Laryngeal tumour Upper airway obstruction **! Remember:** Alert medical staff as airway is at risk of compromise

HAZARD

If you auscultate and hear nothing, a "silent" chest, it may mean the patient is unable to move air at all. This is a medical emergency and you need to get medical assistance immediately!

NATIONAL EARLY WARNING SCORES (NEWS2 2017)[2]

The scores are:
1. To highlight changes in the physiologic status of the patient with routine observations.
2. To empower staff to act and seek additional support for patients whose status has deteriorated (Table 2.14).

A significant change in score of 3 in one or more categories, or 5 and over in total (depending on the scoring system) can trigger outreach or critical care support – see local policy for referral criteria.

A patient who has not reached the trigger score—does not preclude a call for help or advice.

TABLE 2.14   NATIONAL EARLY WARNING SCORE 2

PHYSIOLOGIC PARAMETER	SCORE						
	3	2	1	0	1	2	3
Respiration rate (per minute)	≤8		9–11	12–20		21–24	≥25
SpO$_2$ scale 1 (%)	≤91	92–93	94–95	≥96			
SpO$_2$ scale 2 (%)	≤83	84–85	86–87	88–92 ≥93 on air	93–94 on oxygen	95–96 on oxygen	≥97 on oxygen
Air or oxygen?		Oxygen		Air			
Systolic blood pressure (mmHg)	≤90	91–100	101–110	111–219			≥220
Pulse (per minute)	≤40		41–50	51–90	91–110	111–130	≥131
Consciousness				Alert			CVPU
Temperature (°C)	≤35.0		35.1–36.0	36.1–38.0	38.1–39.0	≥39.1	

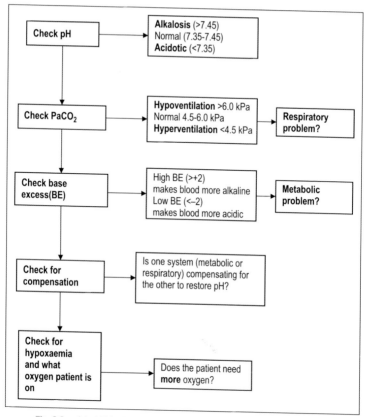

Fig. 2.3 • Arterial blood gas analysis. $PaCO_2$, Partial pressure of carbon dioxide.

THINGS CHANGE!

Your patient may improve or deteriorate during assessment or treatment. This does not necessarily reflect badly on your treatment. Go back to the beginning (ABC) to ensure patient safety.

POTENTIAL PHYSIOTHERAPY PROBLEM LIST

Your goal during assessment is to find out whether the patient has (or is at risk of developing) one or more of the following four physiotherapy problems:

- Sputum retention (see Chapter 5)
- Volume loss (see Chapter 6)
- Increased work of breathing (see Chapter 7)
- Respiratory failure (see Chapter 8)

Management of each of these problems is summarised in these chapters and the decision-making process, shown in Fig. 2.2.

References

1. https://www.resus.org.uk/resuscitation-guidelines/abcde-approach/.
2. Royal College of Physicians. National Early Warning Score (NEWS) 2: Standardising the assessment of acute-illness severity in the NHS. Updated report of a working party. London: RCP, 2017. Available from: https://www.rcplondon.ac.uk/projects/outputs/national-early-warning-score-news-2.

CHAPTER 3

PAEDIATRIC SPECIFICS

Ellie Melkuhn

PAEDIATRIC CONSENT

Gaining and documenting consent, before assessment and treatment, in children is a more complex process. There are four common situations:

1. Children who lack capacity—this is a child who is too young or does not have the ability to understand the implications of refusing or agreeing to a treatment. Here, a person with parental responsibility may give consent on a child's behalf.
2. Children where parents are absent—when parents are not available to provide consent, the medical professional should consider what is in the child's best interests and then act appropriately.
3. Children under the age of 16 years with capacity—a child is 'Gillick Competent' if they demonstrate sufficient maturity and understanding to comprehend the implications of the intervention; including risks and alternative courses of action. These children are legally allowed to consent to interventions when their parents are absent, or if the parents refuse. If the child is refusing treatment however, the parents can override this and consent to treatment.
4. Children over the age of 16 years with capacity—these patients are permitted by law to consent or deny treatment without parental agreement.

The way in which consent or not was obtained should always be clearly documented in the notes. For further information refer to CSP information paper: Consent and Physiotherapy Practice 2016.

SAFEGUARDING

Safeguarding is every professionals' responsibility regardless of the brevity of time spent with the child.

PAEDIATRIC ANATOMY AND PHYSIOLOGY

	ANATOMIC/ PHYSIOLOGIC DIFFERENCE	CONSEQUENCE FOR PHYSIOTHERAPY ASSESSMENT OR TREATMENT
Upper airway	Most infants are preferential nose breathers until 4–5 months old	A small amount of nasal secretions can affect a patient's work of breathing. Start your assessment by reviewing the airway, as simple NP suction may resolve respiratory distress
	Nasal airways are smaller and prone to blockage	
	Larynx is higher enabling simultaneous breathing and sucking up to 4 months	A child with a partially occluded airway will struggle to feed. Lack of feeding is a recognised sign of respiratory distress. Conversely, if a patient is feeding well and smiling, you do not need to be acutely worried about their respiratory function
	Tonsils, adenoids and tongue are comparatively large	An upper respiratory tract infection can significantly affect airway patency and respiratory function. It does not respond to physiotherapy intervention
	Mucosa are easily damaged	Ensure you are using appropriate suction catheter size, suction pressure and correct technique when performing suction, as it is easy to cause bleeding and trauma

Continued

PAEDIATRIC ANATOMY AND PHYSIOLOGY—cont'd

	ANATOMIC/ PHYSIOLOGIC DIFFERENCE	CONSEQUENCE FOR PHYSIOTHERAPY ASSESSMENT OR TREATMENT
Lower respiratory tract airways	Airways in children are significantly smaller	A small amount of secretions or inflammation can affect work of breathing. You may require higher ventilation pressures than expected to combat airway resistance
	A small amount of oedema can cause significant airway narrowing (up to 80%)	Removal of secretions that are further narrowing airways can improve respiratory function
	Airways have a high resistance to airflow	
	Tracheal rings primarily cartilage, softer than in adults	Large negative pressure from diaphragmatic pull during episodes of increased work of breathing can results in tracheal narrowing, further exacerbating work of breathing
Bronchial structure	Children have more mucous glands (17 per/mm in comparison to adults 1 per/mm)	Children make more mucous and are less able to remove it from their lungs They are more likely to need assistance from physiotherapists to clear their sputum and respond well to interventions
	Cilia are immature	
Collateral ventilation	Fewer pores of Kohn in infants	Collateral ventilation is less effective making them more prone to atelectasis and volume loss.
	Canals of Lambert absent in under 4 years of age	Treatments that aim to optimise this (such as MHI inspiration holds), are less effective in children

Ribs	Horizontally positioned, rib structure does not allow for increased tidal volumes	Children will not be able to increase their tidal volume to meet respiratory demand. The only mechanism for improving minute volume is to increase respiratory rate Respiratory rate rise is therefore one of the first signs of respiratory distress
	Weak intercostal muscles with minimal fatigue resistant fibres	Intercostal muscles fatigue quickly. Their weakness contributes to the changes in V̇/Q̇ matching in paediatrics (see later), and why children demonstrate intercostal recession as a sign of respiratory distress
	Ribs more cartilaginous	Paediatric ribs respond well to manual techniques. Some advocate vibrations that compress up to 50% of the thoracic space. Because of the cartilaginous nature of the ribs, you are less likely to cause fractures in children (however, check the patient does not have osteopenia of prematurity or low bone density)
Diaphragm	Flat diaphragm works at a mechanical disadvantage	This prevents children from being able to increase tidal volume, making the patient reliant on increasing breathing rate to match respiratory demand Children are more affected by gas trapping, which further flattens the diaphragm
	Few fatigue resistant fibres (only 25% are slow twitch fibres, in comparison to 50% of adult diaphragm)	Tires quickly when working hard and may develop respiratory failure quicker than an adult
	Main muscle of ventilation	Because of weakness of intercostal and other accessory muscles Children with neuromuscular disorders affecting their diaphragm will have a bigger impact on their respiratory function
	Abdominal organs are relatively large	Supine positioning will disadvantage the diaphragm. A quick way to improve a child's work of breathing and increase basal expansion is to position them in full side lying, or prone; this offloads the abdominal organs and reduces their impact on the respiratory system

Continued

PAEDIATRIC ANATOMY AND PHYSIOLOGY—cont'd

	ANATOMIC/ PHYSIOLOGIC DIFFERENCE	CONSEQUENCE FOR PHYSIOTHERAPY ASSESSMENT OR TREATMENT
Metabolic rate	Children have a higher metabolic rate	They have higher oxygen requirements and deteriorate faster
	Increased oxygen demand	They use up their oxygen reserves quickly and become physiologically unstable in low oxygen states
Ventilation/ perfusion	Nondependent lung is preferentially ventilated	Because of cartilaginous ribs and weak intercostal muscles, the dependent lung does not ventilate effectively. The lung with less gravitational or positional disadvantage will ventilate best Children preferentially ventilate their upper lobes
	In small infants, closing volume exceeds the functional residual capacity	In dependent areas, lung collapse may occur during normal tidal breathing. This increases risk of atelectasis and is one of the reasons why they respond well to PEEP/ CPAP
	Perfusion is the same as adults	Perfusion will be best in gravity dependent areas, which often results in a $\dot{V}/\dot{Q}$ mismatch when positioning for postural drainage
	Hypoxia triggers vasoconstriction (hyperoxia results in vasodilation)	Lung areas with poor ventilation will have automatically reduced perfusion Profound hypoxia will lead to vasoconstriction, and ultimately bradycardia because of low oxygen delivery to cardiac muscle

Sleep	Neonates may sleep for up to 20 hours a day. Some 80% of this time may be REM sleep (rapid eye movement/dreaming)	The amount of time they sleep will affect treatment timings and respiratory function
	Inhibition of smooth muscle during REM sleep (affects the intercostal muscles)	Paediatric patients are more likely to have apnoea when sleeping. They may drop into their closing volume on exhalation, resulting in atelectasis
	FRC is reduced during sleep	
	Loss of laryngeal muscle tone results in the child creating greater auto-PEEP	This helps prevent the causes of aforementioned atelectasis
Heart	Greater percentage of connective tissue, and less contractile tissue	Unable to increase stroke volume output so reliant on increasing HR to increase cardiac output.
	The heart is more susceptible to acidosis, hypoglycaemia, low calcium and anaemia	Children are less physiologically tolerant to these and more likely to have CVS instability because of them
	Takes up proportionally more space in the rib cage (1/2 of total space in comparison to 1/3 in adults)	Cardiomegaly can cause bronchial compression leading to LL collapse (left is more vulnerable than R). Be aware of this anatomic difference when analysing chest x-rays

Continued

PAEDIATRIC ANATOMY AND PHYSIOLOGY—cont'd

	ANATOMIC/ PHYSIOLOGIC DIFFERENCE	CONSEQUENCE FOR PHYSIOTHERAPY ASSESSMENT OR TREATMENT
General	Larger skin surface area to body mass ratio	Children will lose temperature quickly when uncovered. Be mindful of this when assessing and treating
	The neonatal respiratory centre is immature causing irregular breathing patterns and apnoea	Be aware of this when evaluating work of breathing in a newborn. This is not a specific sign of respiratory distress
	Gastrooesophageal reflux is physiologically normal in neonates	Take note of feed times, as this will affect treatment timing. Children are more likely to vomit with physiotherapy than adults. Aspiration is a common cause of respiratory distress and responds well to physiotherapy
	Vagal reflexes are more sensitive in neonates	A small amount of airway stimulation can result in a large parasympathetic response, such as sudden desaturation and bradycardia.

CPAP, Continuous positive airway pressure; CVS, cardiovascular system; FRC, functional residual capacity; LL, left lung; MHI, manual hyperinflation; NP, nasopharyngeal; PEEP, positive end expiratory pressure; V̇/Q̇, ventilation/perfusion.

SIGNS AND SYMPTOMS OF RESPIRATORY DISTRESS IN PAEDIATRIC PATIENTS

SIGN/SYMPTOM	CAUSE
Weak cry	Unable to take a large breath in or expel with enough force to make a normal cry
Grunting	Breathing out against a slightly closed glottis to increased auto-PEEP, to improve FRC and reduce work of breathing
Tachypnoea	Unable to increase tidal volume, they need to increase their respiratory rate to increase minute ventilation
Tracheal tug	Caused by the negative pressure generated by the pull of the diaphragm during inspiration. This affects the soft tissues of the thorax and results in them being pulled inwards
Sternal recession	
Subcostal recession	
Intercostal recession	
Nasal flaring	Dilation of the nares to increase the diameter of the airway and decrease resistance
Head bobbing	Because of the activation of accessory muscles (sternocleidomastoid), against weak core stability/ posterior neck muscles
Stridor	On inspiration caused by narrowing of a floppy airway because of the pull of the diaphragm
Tachycardia	Infants cannot increase stroke volume to increase cardiac output. They increase their heart rate to increase oxygen delivery to the body
Hypoxia	Because of a failure to get adequate oxygen supply into the bloodstream
Hypercarbia	Because of failure to get adequate carbon dioxide clearance
Lethargy	Because of reduced PaO_2 and increasing $PaCO_2$
Bradycardia	Poor oxygenation of cardiac muscle because of the inability to meet metabolic demand
Apnoea	Reduce oxygenation and fewer fatigue resistant fibres in respiratory muscles results in absence of respiratory effort

FRC, functional residual capacity; $PaCO_2$, partial pressure of carbon dioxide; PaO_2, partial pressure of oxygen; PEEP, positive end expiratory pressure.

Safeguarding is defined as:
- Protecting children from maltreatment
- Preventing impairment of childrens' health and development
- Ensuring children grow up in circumstances consistent with the provision of safe and effective care
- Taking action to enable all children to have the best outcomes

Every local authority and National Health Services Trust has a Child Protection (Safeguarding Children) policy, which must be adhered to. You must familiarise yourself with local policy, which should include who to inform and where to document concerns.

Normal Observation Values

The anatomic and physiologic differences between adults and children results in different expected values for cardiovascular and respiratory observations. You need to know what the normal values/range is for the patient's age. Without knowledge of normal you cannot recognise abnormal.

Respiratory Rate

Variations to respiratory rate because of:
- Horizontally positioned ribs
- Weak intercostal muscles
- Flat diaphragm
- Higher metabolic rate
- Increased oxygen demand

This changes as children grow and mature

AGE (YEARS)	RESPIRATORY RATE (BREATHS PER MINUTE)
<1	30–40
1–2	26–34
2–5	24–30
5–12	20–24
>12	12–20

Heart rate

Variations to heart rate (HR) because of:

- Greater percentage of connective tissue, and less contractile tissue
- Unable to increase stroke volume output
- Reliance on increasing HR to improve cardiac output
  This changes as children grow and mature

AGE	HEART RATE (BEATS PER MINUTE)
Newborn–3 months	85–205
2 months–2 years	100–180
2–10 years	60–140
>10 years	60–100

Blood pressure

Blood pressure (BP) is affected by HR, stroke volume and systemic vascular resistance. This changes as children grow and mature.

Variations to BP as child ages and grows:

- HR reduces
- Stroke volume increases
- Systemic vascular resistance increases

AGE	MEAN BLOOD PRESSURE MMHG (5TH CENTILE)	MEAN BLOOD PRESSURE MMHG (50TH CENTILE)
0–1 Month	35	45
1–12 Months	40	55
1–10 Years	40+ (1.5 x age in years)	55+ (1.5 x age in years)
15 Years	65	80

Mean BP values are provided as this is a more accurate measure of tissue perfusion in shock state situations.

Observation norm values from Paediatric Immediate Life Support 3rd Edition, Published by the Resuscitation Council UK.

CHEST X-RAY INTERPRETATION

Stephen Harden

This chapter describes the x-ray appearance of common conditions that you will see when on call. As the majority of patients requiring emergency physiotherapy are short of breath or have suboptimal gas exchange, only abnormalities of the lungs and pleural spaces are demonstrated. Only frontal x-rays (posteroanterior [PA] and anteroposterior [AP]) are used, as these are the ones that you to interpret.

Remember that a perfect chest x-ray (CXR; Fig. 4.1) requires correct patient positioning and the correct x-ray dose. Deficiency in any of these results in a suboptimal x-ray and may produce appearances that simulate lung pathology.

NORMAL LOBAR ANATOMY

* The right lung contains three lobes, upper (RUL), middle (RML) and lower (RLL) (Fig. 4.2A and B).
* On the right side, the oblique fissure separates the RUL from the RLL above the horizontal fissure, and the RML from the RLL below it.
* The horizontal fissure separates the RUL from the RML.

Remember!

When looking at a frontal CXR:
* RUL is at the top, above the horizontal fissure
* RML is at the base anteriorly below the horizontal fissure
* RLL is posterior

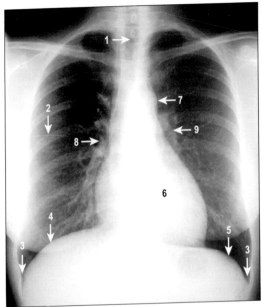

Fig. 4.1 • Normal chest x-ray. Key: 1, trachea; 2, horizontal fissure; 3, costophrenic angle; 4, right hemidiaphragm; 5, left hemidiaphragm; 6, heart shadow; 7, aortic arch; 8, right hilum; 9, left hilum.

- The left lung consists of two lobes, upper (LUL) and lower (LLL) (Fig. 4.2C). The lingula is the most inferior part of the LUL.
- The oblique fissure on the left side separates the LUL and LLL.

Remember!

The LUL is anterior and the LLL is posterior.

For descriptive purposes, the lungs on the CXR are divided into thirds or zones (Fig. 4.2D):

- Upper zone
- Mid-zone
- Lower zone.

These are *not* anatomic divisions. For example, the apex of the lower lobe on each side is in the mid-zone.

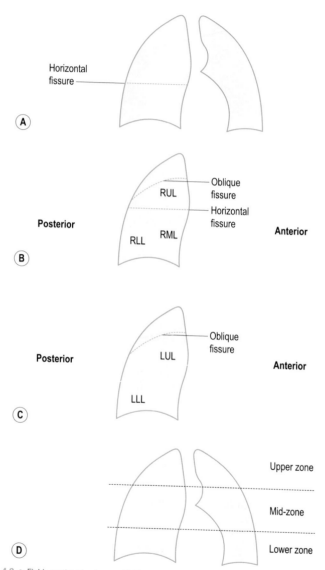

Fig. 4.2 • Fields on the chest x-ray. (A) Frontal plane. (B) Right lung, lateral. (C) Left lung, lateral. (D) Lung field zones. *LLL*, Lower left lung; *LUL*, left upper lung; *RLL*, right lower lung; *RML*, right middle lung; *RUL*, right upper lung.

HOW TO INTERPRET ABNORMALITIES IN THE LUNG FIELDS ON THE CHEST X-RAY

Essentially, these areas are abnormal because they appear either too white or too black.

Too White
The most common causes are:
- Collapse or atelectasis
- Consolidation
- Pleural effusion
- Pulmonary oedema

Too black
The most important causes are:
- Pneumothorax
- Chronic obstructive pulmonary disease (COPD).

ATELECTASIS/COLLAPSE

Atelectasis or collapse refers to an area of lung which is airless and the lung collapses in this region. Atelectasis may involve small areas, an entire lobe or even an entire lung.

The CXR will show a loss of lung volume, the lung field smaller than expected. Other structures may move to fill up the space, so there may be:
- Shift of the mediastinal structures, such as the heart or trachea
- Elevation of the hemidiaphragm compared with the other side

The area of collapsed lung appears as a white or 'dense' area and this represents airless lung tissue. When this affects a small volume of the lung, the appearance is of a white line and this is often seen at the lung bases in postoperative patients. When a whole lobe collapses, each produces a specific appearance (see Fig. 4.3–4.7).

When a whole lung collapses, there is increased density of the entire hemithorax (Figs. 4.8 and 4.9). This appearance is sometimes called a *white-out*, although there are other causes for this. A pneumonectomy is in effect an extreme form of complete lung collapse and so will look the same on CXR, but you may see rib irregularity marking the site of the thoracotomy.

TABLE 4.1   APPEARANCE OF LOBAR COLLAPSE

LOBE COLLAPSE	PRESENTATION
RUL collapse	• There is increased density high in the right lung down to the horizontal fissure • This fissure swings upwards and can adopt an almost vertical position (Fig. 4.3)
RML collapse	• The RML collapses down against the right heart border, which becomes indistinct (Fig. 4.4) • The right heart border is clearly seen on a normal CXR because it lies adjacent to the air-filled middle lobe
RLL collapse	• There is a triangular density low in the right lung, but the right heart border can still be clearly seen (Fig. 4.5)
LUL collapse	• The left lung is slightly whiter than the right • The LUL is anterior and so collapses against the anterior chest wall. Thus you see air in the LLL through the dense collapsed LUL (Fig. 4.6)
LLL collapse	• A triangular density is seen behind the heart (Fig. 4.7) • The part of the heart shadow to the left of the spine is whiter than that to the right of the spine

CXR, Chest x-ray; *LLL*, left lower lobe; *LUL*, left upper lobe; *RLL*, right lower lobe; *RML*, right middle lobe; *RUL*, right upper lobe.

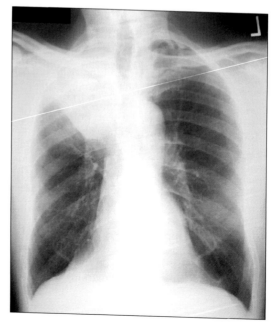

Fig. 4.3 • Right upper lobe collapse. The horizontal fissure is now oriented obliquely. The trachea is deviated to the right, which is evidence of mediastinal shift.

Fig. 4.4 • Right middle lobe collapse. The right heart border is indistinct and there is a vague white appearance to the adjacent lung.

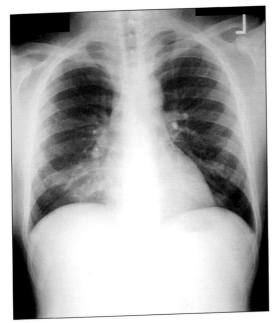

Fig. 4.5 • Right lower lobe collapse. There is abnormal whiteness with a straight outer border (*arrow*) low in the right lung. The right heart border is still visible.

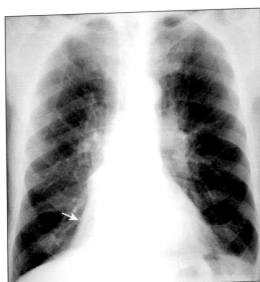

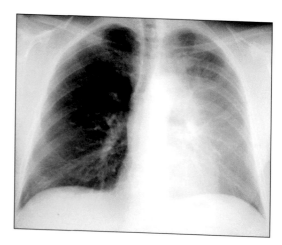

Fig. 4.6 • Left upper lobe collapse. There is a hazy increased whiteness over the left hemithorax. The left heart border is indistinct.

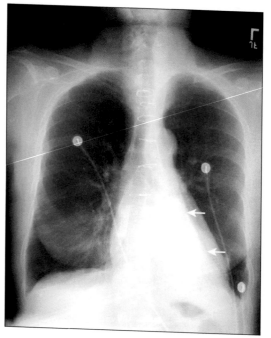

Fig. 4.7 • Left lower lobe collapse. Increased whiteness is seen behind the heart with a straight outer edge (*arrows*).

Fig. 4.8 • Left lung collapse. There is abnormal whiteness over the left hemithorax. The heart is shifted to the left within the abnormal area.

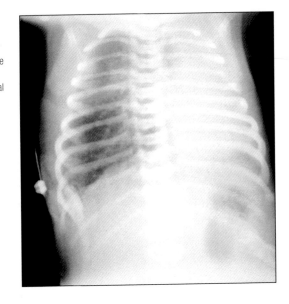

Fig. 4.9 • Pneumonectomy. Abnormal whiteness is seen in the left hemithorax. The trachea and heart are shifted to the left.

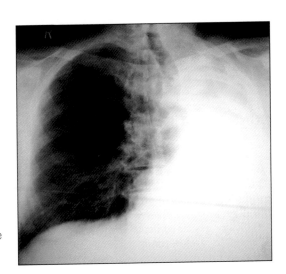

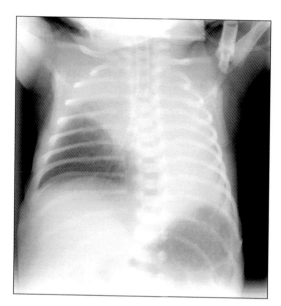

Fig. 4.10 • Collapse of the left lung and right upper lobe. Note the tip of the endotracheal tube, which lies in the right bronchus intermedius.

Remember!

When you see complete collapse of the left lung associated with RUL collapse, in a ventilated patient, always check the position of the endotracheal tube. If the tube has been advanced down the right main bronchus, then only the RML and RLL will be aerated (Fig. 4.10).

CONSOLIDATION

Consolidation occurs when air in lung is replaced by fluid. The distribution of this consolidation may be patchy or may affect an entire segment or lobe. The composition of this fluid depends on the cause:

- Infected fluid, as in pneumonia (the most common cause that you will see)
- Saliva or gastric contents, seen in cases of aspiration
- Blood, in cases of traumatic lung contusion
- Serous transudate, seen in alveolar pulmonary oedema

Although the distribution may help to elicit the cause, the radiologic appearance of consolidation is the same for all of these.

Radiologic Appearance

- The **whiteness or shadowing** in the lung is **poorly defined.** It is difficult to see the edges of these areas. The shadowing has been described as 'fluffy' in appearance.
- There is **no loss of volume,** unlike atelectasis, because there is no lung collapse (Fig. 4.11).
- An air **bronchogram** may be seen, particularly when there is extensive consolidation. This is caused by consolidation of lung tissue, adjacent to an air-filled bronchus, which thus stands out as a black tube amid the consolidative shadowing (Fig. 4.12).

Knowledge of lobar anatomy helps to localise consolidation as it does with atelectasis (Fig. 4.13). It is important in terms of how you treat your patient and may also provide clues as to the cause:

- Aspiration tends particularly to affect the right lower lobe when the patient is erect, as the right main and lower lobe bronchi are the most vertical (Fig. 4.14).

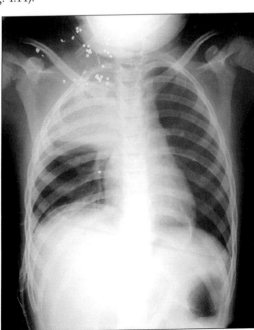

Fig. 4.11 • Traumatic consolidation of the right upper lobe. There is abnormal whiteness in the right upper lobe. The horizontal fissure is in its normal position, so there is no volume loss. Note the shrapnel in the soft tissues.

- Aspiration is particularly seen in the apical segments of the lower lobes when the patient is supine, as these bronchi are directed posteriorly and are thus the most dependent in a patient lying flat.
- Lung contusion tends to occur in the setting of trauma so there may be skin bruising, and you may see rib fractures on the CXR (Fig. 4.15).

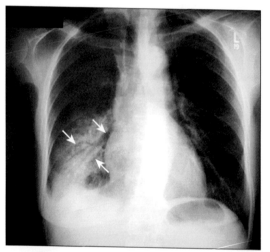

Fig. 4.12 • Right lower lobe consolidation. The abnormal whiteness in the right lower and mid-zones is poorly defined and 'fluffy'. There is a trident-shaped lucency, which is an air broncho-gram (*arrows*). The right heart border remains visible.

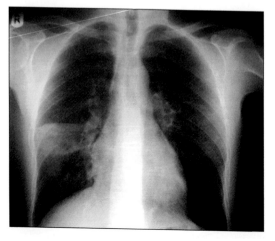

Fig. 4.13 • Middle lobe consolidation. The poorly defined 'fluffy' increased whiteness abuts the horizontal fissure and there is no volume loss.

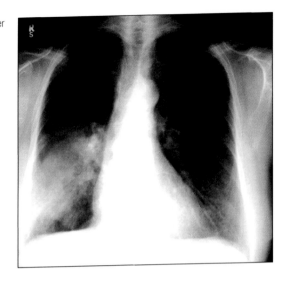

Fig. 4.14 • Right lower lobe consolidation. The upper limit of this abnormal whiteness shows the location of the apical segment of the right lower lobe, which is in the mid-zone.

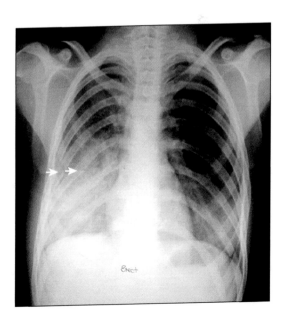

Fig. 4.15 • Traumatic right lower lobe con-solidation. Note the rib fractures (*arrows*).

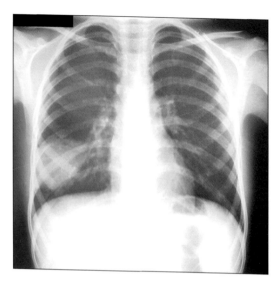

Fig. 4.16 • Round pneumonia. The rounded patchy white area in the right lower zone represents consolidation.

- In alveolar pulmonary oedema, the consolidation appearance tends to be situated in the mid-zones around the hila.

In children, infective consolidation is often circular in shape. This is termed a *round pneumonia* (Fig. 4.16).

Remember!

In real life, consolidation and atelectasis commonly occur together, but by analysing the abnormal white areas on the CXR, you will find that one of these tends to predominate and thus is probably the most important when it comes to treating the patient.

PLEURAL EFFUSION

This refers to fluid in the pleural space. It occupies the dependent part of the pleural space because of gravity, so when the patient is erect or semi-erect, it occupies the lower zone on CXR initially. However, if the patient is supine, it occupies the posterior surface of the pleural space.

Radiologic Appearance

The characteristic feature of the abnormal whiteness of a pleural effusion is that its density is **uniform** throughout. It is not patchy.

Most patients that you will see will have their x-rays taken erect or semi-erect:

- A small effusion presents as blunting of the costophrenic angle, the region on the CXR between the hemidiaphragm and the chest wall.
- In a moderate-sized effusion, the top of the fluid is seen as a horizontal line and there is a meniscus at the point where the fluid touches the chest wall. The hemidiaphragm is obscured (Fig. 4.17).
- With a very large effusion, there may be shift of the mediastinum away from the side of the effusion. A large effusion is another cause for a 'white-out' appearance but the position of the mediastinum tells you if it is caused by atelectasis or effusion (Fig. 4.18).

If the patient is supine, the fluid adopts a posterior location. Thus there will be a generalised increased whiteness of the lung field. The lung can still be seen and is effectively being viewed through a thin layer of fluid.

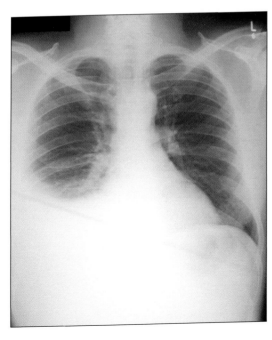

Fig. 4.17 • Right pleural effusion. There is uniform whiteness at the base of the right hemithorax with a horizontal upper surface and a meniscus seen at the chest wall.

PULMONARY OEDEMA

The majority of cases are caused by left ventricular failure. The features are as follows:

- The heart is usually enlarged.
- There may be consolidation around the hila as described earlier (Fig. 4.19).

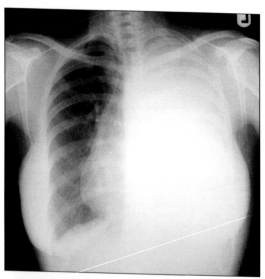

Fig. 4.18 • Left pleural effusion. There is uniform whiteness over the left hemithorax and the heart and mediastinum are displaced to the right. Thus there is 'too much volume' on the left because of a massive pleural effusion.

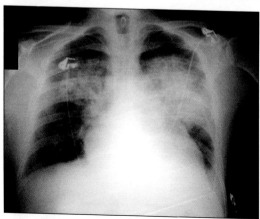

Fig. 4.19 • Heart failure and alveolar pulmonary oedema. The heart is enlarged and there is bilateral consolidation around the hila, the so-called *bat's wing* appearance. Note the small left pleural effusion.

Fig. 4.20 • Interstitial pulmonary oedema. The heart is enlarged. There is prominence of the upper lobe veins (*arrow*), representing upper lobe blood diversion. Kerley B lines are seen at the right base and there is a small right-sided pleural effusion.

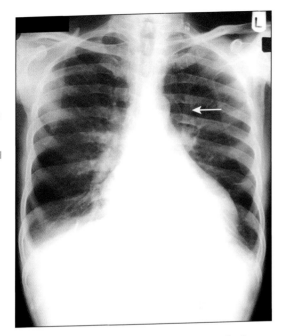

- There may be tiny, thin, horizontal lines, which are seen in the lower zones where the lung touches the chest wall. These are caused by oedema in the lung substance or interstitium rather than the alveoli and are known as Kerley B lines (Figs. 4.20 and 4.21).
- There are large distended veins seen in the upper zones (see Fig. 4.20).
- There may be pleural effusions.

PNEUMOTHORAX

This is an important cause of a lung field appearing too black and refers to air in the pleural space. The features on the CXR are:
- The lung edge is seen as a white line parallel to the chest wall (Fig. 4.22).
- Lung markings do not extend out beyond this white line.
- The area outside this lung edge is blacker than the area inside the line.

A pneumothorax may involve the entire hemithorax and in this case, there will be no lung markings visible at all. In a tension pneumothorax, the air in the pleural space steadily increases and can build

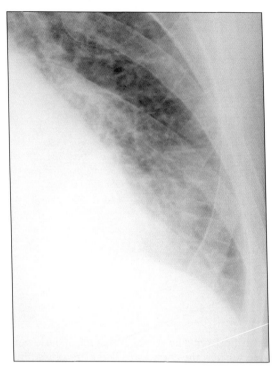

Fig. 4.21 • Kerley B lines. Thin horizontal white lines are seen reaching the pleural surface at the costophrenic angle.

up significant pressure, pushing the mediastinum away towards the opposite side (Fig. 4.23). This can cause cardiac arrest and is thus a surgical emergency.

Hazard

You should not use positive pressure ventilation (e.g., continuous positive airway pressure, intermittent positive pressure breathing or nonivasive ventilation) in a patient with a pneumothorax, as you may turn it into a tension pneumothorax.

Occasionally, the air in the pleural cavity may be located anteriorly, particularly when the patient is supine. This makes it more difficult to see as there may not be a visible lung edge. Be suspicious if the CXR of a ventilated patient shows one lung to be blacker than the other, particularly in the lower zone, and is associated with otherwise unexplained suboptimal gas exchange.

Fig. 4.22 • Right pneumothorax. A black area in the right hemithorax surrounds the right lung, whose edge is clearly seen as a white line (*arrows*). Lung markings do not extend into this black area.

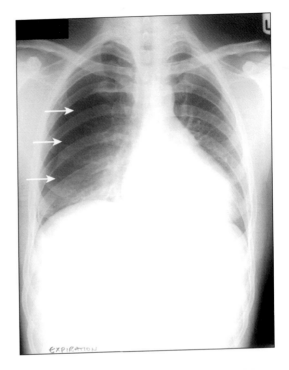

Fig. 4.23 • Left tension pneumothorax. The left hemithorax contains no lung markings at all. The heart and mediastinum are shifted to the right.

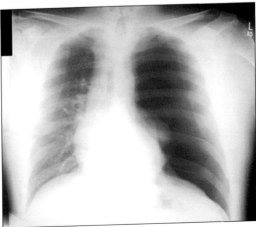

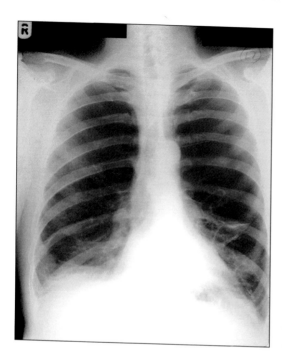

Fig. 4.24 • Chronic obstructive pulmonary disease. Both lungs are blacker than normal, particularly in the upper zones. No lung edge is visible. Close inspection shows lung markings reaching all the way to the pleural surface and chest wall on each side.

CHRONIC OBSTRUCTIVE PULMONARY DISEASE

The lungs appear hyperinflated and blacker in emphysema because of the destruction of lung tissue. Thin-walled sacs or bullae may develop and appear as particularly black areas, often at the top of the lung. In these cases, unlike pneumothorax, there is no visible lung edge and lung markings are seen reaching the chest wall (Fig. 4.24).

Hazard

If you use positive pressure ventilation in these patients, be aware that there is a risk of creating a pneumothorax by rupturing one of the thin-walled bullae. Usually, the benefits to the patient outweigh this small risk, but it is important to discuss this with a doctor.

Acknowledgements

I am grateful to Dr D.J. Delany and Dr I.W. Brown for the use of their extensive film collection and to Dr J.D. Argent for supplying the film of round pneumonia.

Further Reading

Corne, J., Carroll, M., Brown, I., Delany, D., 2002. Chest X-Ray Made Easy, second ed. Churchill Livingstone, London.

CHAPTER 5

MANAGEMENT OF SPUTUM RETENTION

Sandy Thomas, Mary Ann Broad and Matthew J. Quint

Sputum is the material expectorated (coughed up) and is normally mucus and saliva but can also contain pus, blood, epithelial cells, and bacteria/viruses. (Patients may refer to this as spit, phlegm, mucus or gob for example).

DEFINITION

Sputum retention is when patients cannot clear sputum adequately, either independently or with physiotherapy support. This may contribute to acute problems, such as airway obstruction, respiratory infections, increased work of breathing, ventilation/perfusion ($\dot{V}/\dot{Q}$) mismatch and respiratory failure.

When assessment findings suggest sputum retention, particularly if it is causing any of the aforementioned problems, it is important to select the most effective airway clearance technique(s) with the least adverse effects for the patient. Sputum retention is a medical emergency when it causes a blockage of a major airway and/or results in respiratory failure.

CLINICAL SIGNS/ASSESSMENT

Sputum retention is not always evident from auscultation or palpation, so it is important to look for 'clues' which may suggest this problem. Be careful assessing the patient who is breathing shallowly as the signs and symptoms (Table 5.1) may not be easily found.

TABLE 5.1	SIGNS AND SYMPTOMS OF SPUTUM RETENTION
Audible noise at mouth	Crackles, bubbling sounds or coarse wheezing at the mouth during coughing, deep breathing or forced expiration
Palpation	Crackles may be felt directly over the affected area as a popping sensation under the skin
Auscultation	Crackles or wheezes (which may clear after coughing)
Coughing	Frequent attempts at coughing in an awake patient where sputum is in the main airways
History	Patient says it is difficult to clear secretions. Past medical history may indicate a condition associated with sputum, like bronchiectasis or chronic obstructive pulmonary disease (COPD)
Sputum	Look for evidence that sputum is infected or thick/sticky, as it is more likely to be retained
Chest x-ray	Sputum plugging in an airway may lead to atelectasis/lobar collapse. Patchy consolidation may also be seen
Ventilator display (for ventilated patients)	Patients may present with increased airway pressure and/or reduced tidal volumes. The waveforms may have jagged edges indicating airway obstruction. (See critical care–Chapter 13 for management of ventilated patients)

TYPES OF SPUTUM		
Type	Colour	Significance
Mucoid	Clear, white or grey	Usually normal
Mucopurulent	From yellow to green/green brown	Infection attracts neutrophils forming pus in the sputum. Colour depends on bacteria involved
Rusty	Orange brown	Haemoglobin from red blood cells is broken down causing a rusty coloured sputum. Seen after consolidation in pneumonia
Bloody sputum	Red/dark red—blood stained. Blood may be fresh (bright red) or older (darker red)	Haemoptysis from damaged blood vessels in the respiratory tract. Associated with acute trauma or disease including cystic fibrosis or bronchiectasis
Frothy sputum	White or pink	Suggests pulmonary oedema usually associated with heart failure

Sputum retention can cause secondary problems (Table 5.2) but bear in mind these could also be for other reasons.

TABLE 5.2	ADDITIONAL SIGNS AND SYMPTOMS OF SECONDARY PROBLEMS THAT MAY BE CAUSED BY SPUTUM RETENTION
Airway obstruction	Would you recognise this? (See ABC approach in Assessment–Chapter 2)
Respiratory infection	Pyrexia, increased RR, tachycardia increased WBC count and CRP
Increased work of breathing	Increased use of accessory muscles, increased RR, tachycardia, fatigue (see Work of breathing–Chapter 7)
Respiratory failure	Reduced P_aO_2 or SpO_2, increased $PaCO_2$ (see Respiratory failure–Chapter 8)

ABC, Airway, breathing, circulation; *CRP*, C-reactive protein; *PaCO$_2$*, partial pressure of carbon dioxide; *PaO$_2$*, partial pressure of oxygen; *SpO$_2$*, pulse oximetry; *RR*, respiratory rate, *WBC*, white blood cell.

CAUSES OF SPUTUM RETENTION

Impaired mucociliary clearance, excessive mucus secretion, impaired cough, or aspiration may all cause sputum retention.

Aspiration of food, stomach contents or pharyngeal secretions into the airways is a common cause of sputum retention in the elderly, those with altered bulbar function or reduced levels of consciousness.

Impaired mucociliary clearance may be caused by:
- Increased volume of secretions produced by the goblet cells
- Increased viscosity of secretions because of dehydration, infection, or abnormal secretion (e.g., cystic fibrosis)
- Paralysis of cilia because of smoking, general anaesthetic, reduced fluid intake or dry oxygen therapy
- Damaged airways (e.g., bronchiectasis)
- Intubation (presence of artificial airway)

Impaired cough and/or reduced expiratory flow rates may be caused by:

- Fatigue
- Breathlessness
- Immobility
- Muscle weakness or paralysis
- Low lung volumes
- Pain
- Reduced level of consciousness related to anaesthesia, analgesia or pathology

Interventions

You have lots of options for airway clearance techniques, so select the most appropriate for the patient. You may need to try several methods, monitoring throughout, to establish which is most effective, and this may change on successive visits.

Initial Considerations

Table 5.3 highlights management strategies requiring joint decision making/liaison with medical/nursing staff to optimally manage the patient with sputum retention.

AIRWAY CLEARANCE TOOLBOX

Table 5.4 suggests a systematic way to consider physiotherapy interventions in spontaneously breathing (nonintubated) patients.

Table 5.5 suggests interventions for ventilated patients.

For details on treatments see Chapter 9.

Many treatments work well when used in combination, for example, active cycle breathing technique (ACBT) with positioning. **Use your clinical reasoning to select the most appropriate technique(s).**

Modifications for specific groups of patients with sputum retention

- For patients with sputum retention who also have increased work of breathing, see Chapter 7.
- Patients with ineffective cough—moving these patients can help mobilise secretions. Focus on treatments that improve tidal volume, move the patient or augment their cough (e.g., MIE).
- Fatigued patients need their rest—make sure they get it! They also respond well to slow single-handed percussion if manual techniques are indicated.

TABLE 5.3	MEDICAL INTERVENTIONS FOR SPUTUM RETENTION
Hydration	• Systemic hydration is a priority because dehydrated airways have inefficient cilia and this should be managed by encouraging drinking • If the patient is unable to maintain sufficient oral fluid intake discuss the potential need for intravenous fluids with medical staff
Humidification	• Ensure oxygen therapy is delivered with an appropriate humidification system • Cold water humidification systems with wide-bore tubing are often used on wards (bubble through systems using narrow tubing are not considered effective) • Heated systems are often used for intubated and noninvasive ventilation patients. • Heated high flow systems, using a heated cannula to deliver high flow oxygen, may be appropriate for some patients
Nebulised saline	• Saline nebulisers (0.9%) may be used regularly through the day or immediately before active clearance techniques—these require prescription • Hypertonic saline can also be considered in discussion with a prescriber
Bronchodilators	Bronchospasm should be managed before airway clearance—treat the patient after bronchodilators (nebuliser or inhaler)
Pain control	Ensure pain is adequately controlled before beginning treatment—check the patient can take deep breaths/huff and move comfortably. Ask for an analgesia review if necessary
Mucolytic drugs (oral)	Carbocisteine may be useful for patients with copious, thick sputum (e.g., cystic fibrosis, COPD)—it requires prescription

• Patients in pain—see Chapter 10. Remember pain is difficult to assess in sedated patients – liaise with nursing and medical staff
• Patients who are unable to cooperate because of reduced alertness or as part of a disease (e.g., delirium, dementia). Consider consent in this situation, you may need to discuss treatment options with medical and nursing colleagues.

If treatment is appropriate, give clear, concise explanations and reassurance during treatment, minimise distractions and use visual prompts

TABLE 5.4 PHYSIOTHERAPY INTERVENTIONS FOR SPONTANEOUSLY BREATHING/NONINTUBATED PATIENTS

Starting Position	Ensure good position—e.g., sitting upright if possible. Avoid the slumped position
Supported cough	Support any incisions/trauma to chest or abdomen to make cough as effective as possible
ACBT	Try this first in conscious, cooperative patients. Adapt it to your patient's needs extending the breathing control as necessary to allow suitable 'rests'
Mobilise	Move patients where possible—side lying, sitting, standing and walking can help to mobilise sputum if it is safe to do so
Manual techniques	Percussion, shaking and vibrations can be useful for patients with thick secretions who are unable to clear these using ACBT and mobility alone. Can be used with postural drainage if necessary
Positioning (postural drainage)	Side lying is useful when patients have generalised secretions. Specific postural drainage positions can be used if sputum is localised to a lobe or series of lobes. Positions often need to be modified
Positive expiratory pressure (PEP) devices or oscillatory PEP	Can be used for patients with chronic lung disease characterised by sputum retention (e.g., cystic fibrosis, COPD, bronchiectasis)
Autogenic drainage	Only use in the acute situation if the patient knows the technique and both you and they are skilled in its use.
Mechanical insufflation/ exsufflation (MIE)	Use with patients who have ineffective cough caused by primary muscle weakness
Intermittent positive pressure breathing (IPPB)	Useful to improve tidal volumes on inspiration to facilitate expectoration. Note: IPPB modes are available positive pressure devices.
Manual assisted cough	For patients with neurologic compromise, e.g., spinal cord injury (SCI), motor neurone disease, Guillain Barré syndrome. Can be used with MIE
Suction (nasopharyngeal or oral)	Only use if sputum is in central airways, patient is unable to cough effectively, and other methods have been ineffective.

TABLE 5.5	PHYSIOTHERAPY INTERVENTIONS FOR INTUBATED VENTILATED PATIENTS
Humidification	Systemic hydration is managed by total fluids into the patient Heated water humidification systems or saline nebulisers are often incorporated into the ventilator circuit
Manual or ventilator hyperinflation (MHI or VHI)	Use to get air behind secretions, increase expiratory flow rates and simulate cough. May be delivered by the ventilator especially in patients who need high levels of positive end expiratory pressure—always use a manometer in the circuit
Positioning	Use side lying for generalised secretions where possible. Specific postural drainage positions may be indicated where secretions are copious and localised to specific segments. Any changes in position are dependent on cardiovascular and neurologic stability
Manual techniques	Can be used in conjunction with MHI or VHI during the expiratory phase. Use when sputum is tenacious and not cleared effectively with suction or suction and MHI/VHI
Suction	Use after chest physiotherapy and/or when secretions are audible in endotracheal (ET) tube. A rise in peak inspiratory pressure on a ventilator may indicate sputum is present and suction is required
Saline installation	Instilling saline routinely is not evidence based, so you should be guided by local policies. Consider instilling up to 5–10 mL of 0.9% saline before suction for patients with very tenacious secretions causing plugging in conjunction with other physiotherapy techniques Saline installation may be more effective when instilled in the 'opposite' position to the postural drainage position appropriate for the affected segment/lobe—before turning the patient for treatment
Manual insufflation:exsufflation (MIE)	Can be used via ET tube (ETT) or tracheostomy. Consider for patients with poor peak cough flow who cannot move sputum into central airways

- Patients with bronchospasm—link treatments to the time of optimal bronchodilator response. Physiotherapy interventions may aggravate bronchospasm, so avoid repeated huffing and coughing.

SUMMARY

Physiotherapy is crucial in the prevention and management of acute airway obstruction, deteriorating respiratory function and respiratory failure caused by sputum retention.

You can select from a number of different airway clearance techniques and identify the most appropriate treatments for the patient according to the indications, contraindications and resources available.

- Assessment is key to effective management
- Identify the likely causes of sputum retention and refer to appropriate staff where they are not amenable to physiotherapy treatment or require medical/nursing interventions
- Determine which physiotherapy techniques are indicated or contraindicated
- Be prepared to change/adapt techniques for the situation. Your choice must be compatible with your competencies
- Carefully monitor the patient's safety and the effectiveness of your techniques
- Choose simple outcome measures (volume of sputum produced, SpO_2, respiratory rate and auscultation findings)

CHAPTER 6

MANAGEMENT OF VOLUME LOSS

Sandy Thomas and Matthew J. Quint

Understanding lung volumes and how they are affected in illness and disease is essential and can help your clinical reasoning and management decisions. Things that reduce lung volumes may be within the lungs or the surrounding structures and may or may not be amenable to physiotherapy.

Fig. 6.1 shows the different lung volumes.

Volume loss usually occurs when one or both of the following are reduced:

- Inspiratory reserve volume (IRV)
- Functional residual capacity (FRC)

Inspiratory reserve volume is the total volume of air that can be inspired beyond a normal tidal inspiration. It is mainly determined by the length of the ribs and the amount of expansion of the thoracic cage and diaphragm during inspiration. Sufficient inspiratory muscle strength is required to make this expansion. Reduced inspiratory capacity may be caused by reduced thoracic mobility, reduced lung compliance, inspiratory muscle paralysis or significant weakness. Reduced inspiratory capacity also leads to reduced **total lung capacity** (TLC) and **vital capacity** (VC). Resting **tidal volume** (TV) is not always affected, but the ability to increase inspiratory volume, in response to increased activity or increased demand for ventilation, may be significantly reduced. This leads to an increased risk of respiratory failure.

Functional residual capacity is the volume of air that remains in the lung after a normal tidal expiration. It is determined by the balance between the inward recoil of the lungs and the outward recoil of the chest wall, when both inspiratory and expiratory muscles are relaxed. It is reduced when the outward expansion of the chest wall is reduced (e.g., with kyphoscoliosis) or when the inward recoil of the lungs is increased (e.g., with atelectasis). One example of the latter is after abdominal surgery. During expiration, as FRC decreases towards

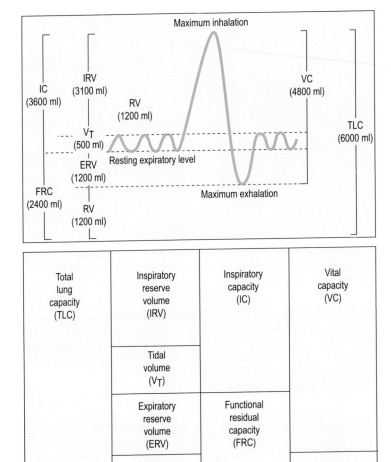

Fig. 6.1 • **Lung volumes** (Reproduced with kind permission from Berne and Levy (2000).)

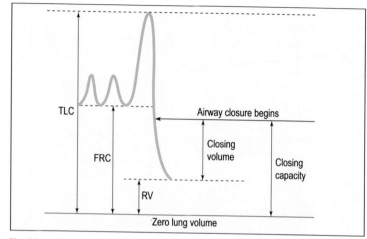

Fig. 6.2 • Closing volumes *FRC*, Functional residual capacity; *RV*, residual volume; *TLC*, total lung capacity. (Reproduced with kind permission from Nunn JF (1999) Nunn's applied respiratory physiology. Oxford: Butterworth-Heinemann.)

residual volume, a point is reached where dependent airways begin to close (closing volume) and remain closed during normal tidal breathing. Gas becomes trapped distal to (beyond) the closed part of the airway and is rapidly absorbed, leading to atelectasis and a reduction in ventilation/perfusion ($\dot{V}/\dot{Q}$) ratios.

This is demonstrated graphically in Fig. 6.2.

Spirometry IRV and FRC can only be measured during laboratory-based tests, so we often do not have access to these measurements. We can however identify reduced lung volumes from clinic-based spirometry tests by looking at the forced vital capacity (FVC) and forced expiratory volume in the first second (FEV_1). These will both be reduced in patients with low lung volumes, but the ratio between the two will be normal (or even increased). Normally, it is possible to expire at least 70% of the FVC in the first second. (FEV_1/FVC ratio is usually >70% or 0.7). A patient with low lung volumes will have a low FVC and a normal FEV_1/FVC ratio. This is known as a ***restrictive pattern***.

Volume loss can be diffuse atelectasis or localised to a specific region of the lung, producing a segmental, lobar or even total lung collapse.

Problems resulting from low lung volumes are reduced compliance, reduced diffusion and reduced V/Q ratios. These cause increased work of breathing breathlessness and reduced exercise tolerance. Type 2 respiratory failure may develop because fatigue leads to an inability to maintain an adequate minute volume.

ASSESSMENT FINDINGS

- Difficulty in taking a deep breath
- Reduced thoracic mobility (bilaterally or unilaterally, may be associated with chest wall deformity or fractures)
- Reduced breath sounds
- Fine crackles possible during inspiration
- Bronchial breathing may be heard over areas of consolidation– (see Auscultation-Chapter 2)
- Chest x-ray (CXR) may demonstrate increased opacity and reduced volume, resulting in shifted structures (see Chapter 4). These may be identified as consolidation, atelectasis, scar tissue, pleural effusion or pneumothorax
- Pain on inspiration
- Reduced exercise tolerance
- Restrictive pattern from spirometry (if available)
- Other observations, such as use of accessory muscles, reduced oxygen saturations, respiratory failure can occur depending on the severity and cause of the volume loss

CAUSES

There are different causes of volume loss and assessment findings vary depending on the cause. It is important to identify causes that are potentially treatable with physiotherapy.

Table 6.1 summarises pathologic mechanisms of volume loss and Table 6.2 links assessment findings to respiratory conditions leading to volume loss.

TABLE 6.1	UNDERLYING PATHOLOGIC MECHANISMS OF VOLUME LOSS
Reduced chest wall/ diaphragm mobility	Chest wall deformity (kyphosis, scoliosis), ankylosing spondylitis, degenerative arthritis, trauma to thorax or abdomen (fractured ribs, abdominal or thoracic surgery) Lung compression: enlarged abdomen (ascites, pregnancy, obesity, constipation) Intrusion of abdominal contents into chest (e.g., diaphragmatic hernia or hiatus hernia) Pleural effusion, mass (e.g., tumour) Pneumothorax Obesity
Reduced lung compliance	Interstitial lung disease Cystic fibrosis Atelectasis (secondary to sputum plugging, causing lobar collapse) Pulmonary oedema Pneumonia, consolidation Adult respiratory distress syndrome (ARDS)
Inspiratory muscle weakness or paralysis	Neuromuscular disease (Guillain Barré, high spinal cord lesions, muscular dystrophy) Reduced respiratory drive (head injury, drugs)

TABLE 6.2	LINKING ASSESSMENT FINDINGS TO DIFFERENT RESPIRATORY PROBLEMS LEADING TO LOW LUNG VOLUMES		
	CHEST WALL OBSERVATION AND PALPATION	CHEST X-RAY	AUSCULTATION
Consolidation	Decreased excursion over affected lobe	Increased opacity air bronchogram Loss of silhouette sign	Bronchial breathing may be heard over consolidated area Coarse crackles sometimes heard when resolving

TABLE 6.2 LINKING ASSESSMENT FINDINGS TO DIFFERENT RESPIRATORY PROBLEMS LEADING TO LOW LUNG VOLUMES—cont'd

	CHEST WALL OBSERVATION AND PALPATION	CHEST X-RAY	AUSCULTATION
Atelectasis	Normal or decreased excursion depending on degree of collapse	Loss of volume, lobar or segmental collapse may cause mediastinal shift towards the volume loss, raised hemidiaphragm, increased opacity and/or white lines at lung bases	Reduced breath sounds in affected areas. Fine Inspiratory crackles may be heard (especially in association with interstitial disease)
Chest trauma	Decreased movement paradoxical breathing (flail segment)	Fractured ribs lung contusion (patchy opacity)	Decreased breath sounds coarse crackles may be heard if airways obstructed
Postabdominal/ thoracic operation	Decreased movement associated with pain or inhibition because of splinting of diaphragm	Reduced lung volume on inspiration	Reduced breath sounds
Pleural effusion	Normal or reduced	Increased opacity with fluid level (position dependent) Possible meniscal sign	Absent breath sounds over effusion – but may hear bronchial breathing at lip of effusion dull to percussion over effusion

Continued

TABLE 6.2	LINKING ASSESSMENT FINDINGS TO DIFFERENT RESPIRATORY PROBLEMS LEADING TO LOW LUNG VOLUMES—cont'd		
	CHEST WALL OBSERVATION AND PALPATION	CHEST X-RAY	AUSCULTATION
Pneumothorax	Reduced movement with possible unilateral hyperinflation on affected side	Blacker appearance Larger apparent volume Pneumothorax will tend to push structures away from it, causing a mediastinal shift Loss of lung markings Edge of collapsed lung visible	Absent breath sounds over pneumothorax Hyperresonant to percussion over area of pneumothorax
ARDS (adult respiratory distress syndrome)	Potentially reduced (not always evident as generally ventilated)	Widespread alveolar shadowing— batwing shadowing	Fine inspiratory crackles

Physiotherapy Strategies to Increase Lung Volumes:

- Controlled mobilisation
- Breathing exercises focusing on thoracic expansion, inspiratory holds and sniffs.
- If using active cycle of breathing technique (ACBT) for sputum retention, minimise forced expiration and emphasise thoracic expansion exercises
- Positioning to optimise expansion
- Positioning to improve length tension relationship of diaphragm
- Continuous positive airway pressure (CPAP) to increase FRC
- Intermittent positive pressure breathing/noninvasive ventilation to increase TV
- Neurofacilitation techniques. If ventilated manual hyperinflation or ventilator hyperinflation (ensure positive end expiratory pressure is maintained throughout)

You must understand why and when to use different techniques and when they may not be appropriate. Table 6.3 summarises potential physiotherapy interventions links this to clinical reasoning.

TABLE 6.3	CLINICAL REASONING LINKED TO PHYSIOTHERAPY INTERVENTIONS FOR VOLUME LOSS
PHYSIOTHERAPY INTERVENTION	CLINICAL REASONING
Mobilising	Get patient up and moving about wherever possible to improve IRV, FRC and TV
Deep breathing exercises	Helps prevent atelectasis if patient unable to mobilise independently/regularly or if necessary, to supplement mobility
Thoracic mobility exercises and mobilisation techniques	If it is possible to improve musculoskeletal function and increase range of motion of thorax Fixed deformities will not respond to physiotherapy, however, postural correction, thoracic mobility exercises and joint mobilisations can sometimes be helpful for joint or soft tissue problems
Pain management	Essential where pain is limiting breathing, coughing and movement—ensure appropriate analgesia
Inspiratory muscle training	If respiratory muscles are weak and can be strengthened. This is a longer-term treatment, useful for patients with chronic respiratory issues
Sputum clearance using manual techniques or ACBT	Where sputum plugging leads to segmental or lobar collapse
Positioning	Upright: Sitting upright in a chair or supported in a forward leaning position achieves higher lung volumes than supine or slumped sitting Side lying: Side lying can be used to free the diaphragm, allowing improved ventilation especially with an enlarged abdomen. Depending on ventilation perfusion matching there may be benefits to having the affected lung either dependent or uppermost

Continued

TABLE 6.3	CLINICAL REASONING LINKED TO PHYSIOTHERAPY INTERVENTIONS FOR VOLUME LOSS—cont'd
PHYSIOTHERAPY INTERVENTION	CLINICAL REASONING
	Prone: Useful for patients with ARDS, widespread atelectasis/collapse in dependent lung areas who are unable to maintain adequate oxygenation. In general, only suitable for patients in critical care and needs appropriate levels of staffing to be able to turn the patient safely. The decision to use prone positioning should be taken by the multidisciplinary team
Postural drainage	Postural drainage may clear secretions, used in conjunction with ACBT and manual techniques
CPAP	Useful for patients with volume loss, who are unable to maintain adequate O_2 saturation even when positioning, mobilising and pain control is optimised

ACBT, Active cycle of breathing technique; *ARDS*, adult respiratory distress syndrome; *CPAP*, continuous positive airways pressure; *FRC*, functional residual capacity; *IRV*, inspiratory reserve volume; *TV*, tidal volume.

SUMMARY

Physiotherapists must identify patients at risk of volume loss because it can lead to breathlessness, reduced exercise tolerance, sputum retention, hypoxemia and ultimately respiratory failure. Physiotherapy assessment identifies the causative factors and clinical reasoning selects the most appropriate interventions for prevention or management.

CHAPTER 7

MANAGEMENT OF WORK OF BREATHING

Matthew J. Quint and Jules Lodge

Patient Story

Bob Head is a 76-year-old male admitted with a 3-day history of increasing breathlessness, temperature and an unproductive cough. He has a previous medical history of chronic obstructive pulmonary disease (COPD) and a kyphoscoliosis.

DEFINITION

The term *work of breathing* (WOB) refers to the energy required by the respiratory muscles to breathe. This is determined by the balance between: the drive to breathe (**demand**), the **load** applied to the respiratory muscles and the efficiency of the respiratory muscles (**capacity**) (Fig. 7.1).

Dyspnoea, breathlessness or shortness of breath is the patient's perception that it is harder work to breathe. Breathlessness may be normal when demand increases, such as during exercise, but it becomes a problem when there is an awareness that the effort made is inappropriate to the amount of air moving in and out and the amount of activity being undertaken.

Dyspnoea may or may not be associated with respiratory failure. The respiratory muscles are normal skeletal muscles and will fatigue if they work too hard. If this is not addressed, the patient will potentially progress to respiratory failure (see Chapter 8). **It is essential that you can identify patients who are fatiguing and at risk of respiratory failure because these patients will need urgent support to reduce their WOB** (Fig. 7.2).

Some patients present with breathlessness related to dysfunctional breathing. Here, it is the drive to breathe that is increased, and may be

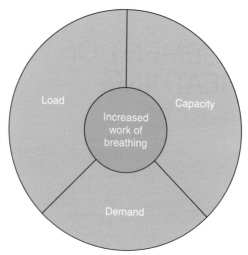

Fig. 7.1 • Schematic representation of the components of work of breathing.

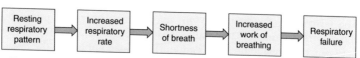

Fig. 7.2 • Schematic representation of the progression as load exceeds respiratory capacity.

excessive, thus the blood gases show signs of hyperventilation (such as decreased $PaCO_2$). It is important you can identify patients who are overbreathing or those for whom anxiety is making breathlessness worse. In this situation, strategies to reduce anxiety are often helpful.

CLINICAL SIGNS/ASSESSMENT

There are a number of simple tools to measure increased WOB. Some are noted by observation from the end of the bed; others require additional equipment or a specific skill requiring support from other colleagues (for example, arterial blood gas sampling) (Tables 7.1 and 7.2).

TABLE 7.1	CLINICAL FEATURES THAT MAY SUGGEST INCREASED WORK OF BREATHING
CLINICAL FEATURES	**RATIONALE**
↑Respiratory rate	The respiratory centre has been stimulated to increase ventilation, because of increased demand or reduced gas exchange
↑ Heart rate	The cardiovascular centre increases the heart rate to improve circulation for oxygen delivery
Mouth breathing	Reduces resistance to air flow to reduce the impact of an increased WOB
Altered respiratory pattern (changes in tidal volume, pursed lipped breathing)	Increased tidal volumes may be more efficient when WOB is increased. Pursed lip breathing prevents airway collapse during expiration and may improve ventilation
Accessory muscle use	Suggests the need for increased respiratory muscle effort to improve ventilation
↓ Oxygen saturation (SpO_2)	Indicates that the increased WOB is significant, and the patient is no longer able to maintain sufficient gas exchange leading to hypoxemia
Deranged arterial blood gases (hypoxia or hypercapnia)	Blood gases become affected when increased WOB delivers ventilation still inadequate to meet demand. It indicates the increased WOB is significant, and the patient is no longer able to maintain an adequate total ventilation (minute volume) to meet the demand for O_2 delivery and CO_2 removal

CAUSE

The key to assessment is to identify the cause of a patient's respiratory distress. The initial screening from the end of the bed may make it clear that the patient is in distress but not the reason. The cause will determine strategies necessary to address the problem. For example, just from the brief history of Mr Head, there are potential causes for his increased WOB.

TABLE 7.2	SIGNS OF HYPOXIA AND HYPERCAPNIA (CO_2 RETENTION)
SIGNS OF HYPOXIA	**SIGNS OF HYPERCAPNIA**
• ↑ respiratory rate • Cough • Shortness of breath • Cyanosis • Cerebral—confusion/anxiety • Cardiac—↑pulse/ ↓pulse / cardiac arrest • Sweating • ↓SpO_2 and ↓partial pressure of oxygen (PaO_2)	• Peripheral vasodilation • Bounding pulse • Tremor of hands • Cerebral—restlessness/irritability confusion/seizure/coma • Cardiac—↑pulse ↑BP/ ↓pulse/ ↓BP/ cardiac arrest • Fatigue • ↑ partial pressure of carbon dioxide ($PaCO_2$)

- He has a chest wall deformity, his kyphoscoliosis changes his respiratory mechanics and infection is likely change the compliance of his lungs, making them stiffer. This changes the **capacity.**
- COPD means there is narrowing of his airways (obstruction) increasing **load.**
- Poor gas exchange from the presumed chest infection leads to hypoxia thus increases **demand.**

These combined increases the effort he needs to make to breathe—thus his WOB has increased.

INTERVENTIONS

If there is:
- Increased load; consider what can be done to reduce the load, for example, positioning, weight loss.
- Reduced capacity; consider how can this be increased—for example, noninvasive ventilation, positive pressure, bronchodilators, nutritional considerations, respiratory muscle training.
- Increased demand; how can this be reduced—for example, relaxation, pain control.

There may also be issues outside your scope of practice. If so, there is nothing wrong with highlighting your concerns to colleagues or other members of the team.

Fig. 7.3 expands Fig. 7.1, giving potential causes of increased WOB for each of those causes.

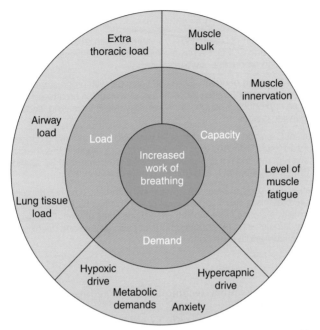

Fig. 7.3 ● Schematic representation of the components of work of breathing and potential underlying causes.

Examining the options, look at the four cases in Table 7.3 and consider whether the patient's increased WOB is caused by one or more of:

Change in load

Change in capacity

Change in demand

Referring back to Fig. 7.1, patient A's breathlessness is likely to be the result of **increased load** coming from both outside and within his thorax. His high BMI will mean there is an increased load on the outside of the chest wall and abdomen. The wheeze and sputum add airflow obstruction increasing load further. Reduction of the load could be achieved by positioning to unload his diaphragm, for example, high side lying. The bronchospasm could be addressed in liaison with colleagues with appropriate bronchodilators, and

TABLE 7.3   FOUR EXAMPLES OF INCREASED WORK OF BREATHING

- Patient A is short of breath. He is 74 years old with a high body mass index (BMI) and COPD. He has a 1-week history of increasing wheeze and a cough productive of white sputum

- Patient B is short of breath. She is 58 years old with progressive multiple sclerosis presenting with a 2-day history of worsening breathlessness and an unproductive cough. Her respiratory rate is increasing, and her expansion is poor.

- Patient C is short of breath. He is 78 years old with underlying congestive cardiac failure, admitted with a 3-day history of increasing breathlessness, a swollen, red and hot right ankle. He has a temperature of $38°$ C and pH 7.35, $PaCO_2$ 4.5, PaO_2 8.4, BE -3 (on 40% O^2)

- Patient D is short of breath. A 28-year-old asthmatic who has become more breathless over the past week or so. This has happened before and normally relates to times when there are pressures at work. She has been dizzy, is breathing apically and reports occasional pins and needles in their fingers and a dry mouth.

simple airway clearance techniques could reduce the obstruction from sputum.

Patient B's underlying **capacity** to meet the load and demand has been exceeded. Increasing the muscle power by strengthening is not an option in the short term. Therefore positioning to optimise her current capacity is key to management. This may allow a degree of rest, as would short-term support of her respiratory muscles with strategies, such as intermittent positive pressure breathing. Improving muscle function with enhanced oxygenation by delivery of prescribed oxygen and optimising ventilation/perfusion ($\dot{V}/\dot{Q}$) matching will also help her (O'Driscoll et al., 2017).

The primary issue with patient C is an increase in respiratory **demand**. There is increased metabolic demand because of both infection (ankle) and his temperature. The relative hypoxia, despite oxygen therapy, is adding to his breathlessness. Adequate oxygen therapy to reverse the hypoxia would be the first priority. Reducing the metabolic demand, by treating the infection, will be down to medical colleagues.

This is different to patient D whose breathlessness is also related to **increased demand**, but this time secondary to anxiety. Reassurance and breathing control can make a significant difference to this person.

BREATHLESSNESS AND ANXIETY

So far, this chapter has focused on the physical and physiologic aspects of increased WOB, however, there is a significant psychological aspect which cannot be ignored which is important to both recognise and address. This interaction is demonstrated in Fig. 7.3.

Although breathlessness is a normal sensation (e.g., when exercising), uncontrollable breathlessness is extremely frightening for anyone. For patients with a chronic respiratory condition, breathlessness can be experienced several times a day with minimal exertion. These patients become extremely anxious about becoming breathless, which further impacts on their breathing—creating a vicious cycle of activity avoidance and deconditioning. It can also become very difficult for this patient group to differentiate between breathlessness because of deconditioning and breathlessness because of exacerbation (Fig. 7.4). This is not always clear cut and once their acute respiratory distress has been appropriately treated the longer-term implications of breathlessness management need to be considered.

Patient Story

Joan is a 68-year-old female admitted with breathlessness, thought to be caused by an exacerbation of her COPD. She is known to have moderate COPD with three admissions for breathlessness in the past month. Each admission has been similar, with worsening symptoms of breathlessness, but no other clinical signs. She lives alone in a bungalow and is starting to find activities of daily living (ADL) difficult.

CLINICAL SIGNS/ASSESSMENT

A calm approach offering practical steps and actions can reassure and will help the patient to bring their breathing under control. These patients show the majority of signs shown in Table 7.1 but these will often be transient and/or episodic. The respiratory rate, pattern and accessory muscle use will often change when the patient becomes more anxious (e.g., just before mobilising), but can be quite normal when settled. This anxiety, about an activity which might cause

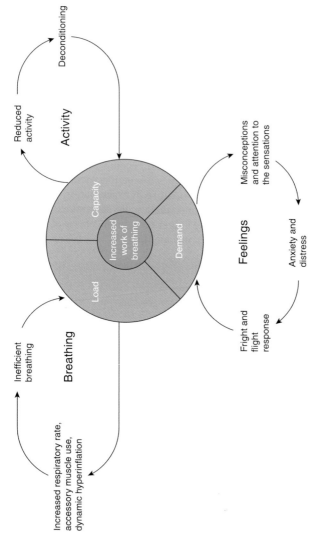

Fig. 7.4 • The interaction between the psychologic and physical aspects of increased work of breathing.

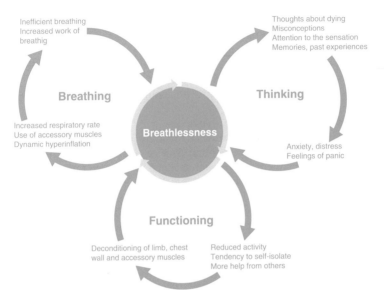

Inefficient breathing
Increased work of
breathig

Thoughts about dying
Misconceptions
Attention to the sensation
Memories, past experiences

Breathing

Thinking

Breathlessness

Increased respiratory rate
Use of accessory muscles
Dynamic hyperinflation

Anxiety, distress
Feelings of panic

Functioning

Deconditioning of limb, chest
wall and accessory muscles

Reduced activity
Tendency to self-isolate
More help from others

Fig. 7.5 The Breathing, Thinking, Functioning clinical model: © Cambridge Breathlessness Intervention Service 2015.

breathlessness, can result in decreased activity and deconditioning. This further increases their sense of respiratory effort. This interaction of load, capacity and demand is shown in Fig. 7.4. The Cambridge Breathlessness Service has developed an evidence based approach (Spathis et al. 2017) to facilitate effective symptom control by focusing on three predominant cognitive and behavioural response to breathlessness (see Fig. 7.5).

CAUSE AND INTERVENTION

When the level of breathlessness is perceived as greater than it should be, the brain sends a high alert message. This results in an increased drive to breathe, increased use of accessory muscles and an increased respiratory rate and effort further alerting the brain and increasing the feeling of breathlessness. This worsening breathlessness then triggers feelings of loss of control and anxiety. Strategies to help the patient bring control to their breathing and empower their abilities may include:

- Borg scale to help with pacing
- Ideas to help with pacing and planning for ADL at home, this may include aids and occupational therapy (OT) assessment
- Box breathing (Treatments, see Chapter 9) to ensure sufficient time for exhalation and avoid breath stacking
- Using a handheld fan to help with cooling the face and increasing sensation of airflow
- Positions to help with breathlessness
- Creating an action plan for when breathlessness occurs
- The Breathlessness Intervention Service (Breathlessness Intervention Service patient information leaflets) and British Lung Foundation (How to manage breathlessness) have some excellent patient focused leaflets covering these topics.

Joan has increased load because of her COPD, reduced capacity because of her weak respiratory and skeletal muscles and increased demand because of anxiety. Addressing this anxiety and providing her with techniques to manage her breathlessness can build her confidence and improve her physical ability. Breaking this cycle will reduce the likelihood of being readmitted. Referrals to community COPD team and pulmonary rehabilitation on discharge would help support her with this.

For some people who have experienced acute or chronic breathlessness, the compensatory respiratory pattern can become normalised. If this persists, they can develop disordered breathing and become more symptomatic.

BREATHING PATTERN DISORDER/DYSFUNCTIONAL BREATHING/HYPERVENTILATION SYNDROME

This is breathing in excess of the body's requirements for an ongoing period of time, which occurs following an acute respiratory event or a stressful situation, after which the individual's normal resting respiratory pattern is not restored. Common symptoms include air hunger, breathlessness, tingling fingers, tight chest, cough, dizziness, sighing/yawning. The symptoms are caused by lower levels of CO_2 in the body because of overbreathing. There is no definitive diagnostic test but there are a few ways of demonstrating it probably is this.

- Complete a Nijmegen questionnaire (Nijmegen Questionnaire)—positive test if scores greater than 23/64.

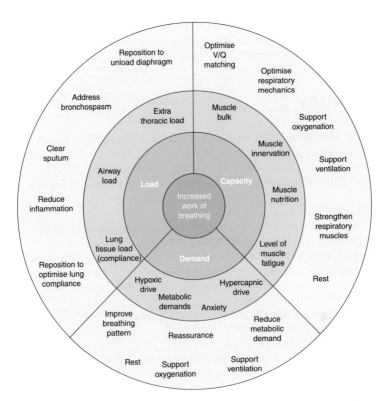

Fig. 7.6 • Components of work of breathing with underlying causes and potential treatment strategies.

- Time a breath hold—if the patient cannot hold for 20 seconds, then this is a likely diagnosis. It is probable if the hold is between 20 to 30 seconds and possible if between 30 to 40 seconds.
- Assess the respiratory rate and pattern—is it fast/slow, shallow/deep, rhythmical/erratic? Are they breathing through their nose/mouth? Is it upper chest/diaphragmatic? Are they taking frequent sighs/yawns? Is there a pause at the end of expiration?
- Do a hyperventilation provocation test (HVPT; HVPT Information) get the patient to breathe rapidly (fast and shallow) for 20 breaths to see if symptoms are provoked.

The first steps in treating this problem would be to encourage nose breathing and teach breathing control exercises. Once identified as having breathing pattern disorder (BPD), a physiotherapist specialising in treating these disorders should be consulted who will deliver an appropriate treatment (possibly as an inpatient) as an outpatient.

SUMMARY

Early identification of increased WOB by a physiotherapist allows the underlying problem to be identified and treated. Early intervention can avoid the patient deteriorating. A summary of the underlying causes linked to strategies to address WOB are presented in Fig. 7.6.

References

O'Driscoll, B.R., Howard, L.S., et al., 2017. BTS Guideline for oxygen use in adults in healthcare and emergency settings. Thorax 72 (Suppl. 1), pi1–pi89.

Spathis A, Booth S, Moffat C, et al. The Breathing, Thinking, Functioning clinical model: a proposal to facilitate evidence-based breathlessness management in chronic respiratory disease. *NPJ Prim Care Respir Med* 2017;27:(1)27). Published 2017 Apr 21. doi:10.1038/s41533-017-0024-z).

Breathlessness Intervention Service breathing, thinking, functioning model. Available from https://www.cuh.nhs.uk/sites/default/files/publications/100079_leaflet_1_the_BTF_approach_v1.pdf.

Breathlessness Intervention Service patient information leaflets. Available from https://www.cuh.nhs.uk/breathlessness-intervention-service-bis/resources/patient-information-leaflets.

How to manage breathlessness information available from https://www.blf.org.uk/support-for-you/breathlessness/how-to-manage-breathlessness.

Nijmegen Questionnaire: https://hgs.uhb.nhs.uk/wp-content/uploads/Nijmegen_Questionnaire.pdf.

HVPT Information. available from https://journals.sagepub.com/doi/pdf/10.1191/1479972306cd116ed.Et qui a nis denimporem iliaerum faccus enderum hario dolum volore

MANAGEMENT OF RESPIRATORY FAILURE

Liz Newton and Matthew J. Quint

Respiratory failure (RF) is a life-threatening problem, which requires prompt and appropriate management from the whole team. This chapter focuses on your role within the team.

DEFINITION

RF results from inadequate gas exchange by the respiratory system, meaning that the arterial oxygen, carbon dioxide or both cannot be kept at normal levels.

TYPE 1 RESPIRATORY FAILURE

Type 1 respiratory failure (T1RF) occurs when the oxygen of arterial blood has a partial pressure of less than 8 KPa (PaO_2 <8 KPa) and a respiratory rate of greater than 24 breaths per minute. The partial pressure of CO_2 (PaCO2) may be normal or low.

Patient Story

Patient A has been admitted to hospital with a history of worsening shortness of breath at rest, cough productive of green sputum and O_2 saturations of 78% on air. He has a background of interstitial pulmonary fibrosis and hypertension.

He is tachypnoeic (rate 42 breaths per minute), he is centrally and peripherally cyanosed. His arterial blood gas (ABG) on O_2 at 10 L/min via nonrebreather reservoir mask on arrival at the emergency department shows pH 7.45, $PaCO_2$ 4.4 KPa, PaO_2 7.9 KPa, HCO_3 25 mmol/L, BE +1

Clinical signs

For clinical signs of hypoxaemia, see Table 7.2 (see Chapter 7 Management of work of breathing). Patients will have increased work of breathing, be tachypnoeic and breathless, finding it difficult to speak in full sentences. They may feel frightened and anxious and appear distressed. They will have positioned themselves (if they are able to do so) to maximise the capacity of their respiratory muscles (e.g., forward lean sitting).

Assessment

To clinically reason the cause of their type 1 RF, make use of the medical notes and confirm the medical diagnosis. Assess their respiratory pattern, auscultation, palpation, thoracic expansion, cough and sputum, presence of haemoptysis, the chest x-ray and/or computed tomography (CT) thorax, full blood count (FBC) results, urea and electrolyte (U&E) results, ABGs results, including lactate, observations, including: pulse oximetry (SpO_2); O_2 requirement; respiratory rate (RR); blood pressure (BP); heart rate (HR); temperature; conscious level (see Chapter 2 Assessment).

You now need to decide whether treatment is appropriate to improve oxygenation and/or WOB.

Ask yourself,

- Does the patient have sputum retention, lobar collapse, volume loss? (See Chapters 5 and 6).
- Is bronchospasm the issue or a pulmonary embolism or pulmonary oedema (requiring medical rather than physiotherapy management)?
- Is there anything you can do to improve the capacity of the respiratory muscles or reduce the load on the respiratory muscles? (See Chapter 7)

Cause (table 8.1)

Patients with type 1 RF initially have the capacity to increase their ventilatory drive in response to hypoxaemia. This can result in respiratory alkalosis as CO_2 is blown off. However, tachypnoea can only be sustained for a certain period of time before the respiratory muscles fatigue (**load** exceeds **capacity** in the environment of increased **demand**.) and the patient starts to hypoventilate and progresses to type 2 RF (T2RF). It is essential you recognise when a patient is tiring and exhibiting signs of T2 RF (see type 2 RF) but an ABG will be required to confirm this.

MANAGEMENT

Your primary goal for Patient A is oxygenate him to achieve his target saturations (94%–98%). This will reduce his ventilatory **demand**. In this case, hypoxaemia (and T1RF) are being caused by $\dot{V}/\dot{Q}$ mismatching because of preexisting lung disease (made worse by sputum retention), and a diffusion defect.

His WOB is affected by **increased load** because of restrictive lung disease (stiff lungs) and sputum retention. **Demand** is raised by

TABLE 8.1 CAUSES OF TYPE 1 RESPIRATORY FAILURE	
CAUSE OF HYPOXAEMIA	EXAMPLES
Ventilation/perfusion mismatch ($\dot{V}/\dot{Q}$ defect).	COPD, pneumonia, asthma, interstitial pulmonary fibrosis, bronchiectasis, pulmonary oedema, pneumothorax, pulmonary embolus, ARDS, lobar collapse.
True pulmonary shunt Does not respond well to simple O_2 therapy, although the addition of a positive pressure (CPAP/PEEP) may help	Large pneumonias/consolidated pneumonitis Large areas of atelectasis ARDS or acute lung injury Small cell lung cancer
Diffusion defects	Thickened respiratory membrane in conditions, such as pulmonary fibrosis and sarcoidosis Reduced lung surface area is most common in emphysema
Hypoventilation of the alveoli This may initially cause hypoxaemia but will progress to type 2 RF if untreated	(See type 2 RF) • Dysfunction of the respiratory centre to drive ventilation • Neuromuscular dysfunction causing weakness (e.g., high spinal injury) • Fatigue of the muscles of ventilation, fixed thoracic cage or worsening of $\dot{V}/\dot{Q}$ mismatch (e.g., severe kyphoscoliosis)

ARDS, Acute respiratory distress syndrome; *COPD*, chronic obstructive pulmonary disease; *CPAP*, continuous positive airway pressure; *PEEP*, positive end expiratory pressure.

hypoxaemia (T1RF). He is managing to maintain a raised RR without CO_2 retention, so his respiratory muscle **capacity** is sufficient. He is at high risk of T2RF however, because his respiratory muscles will fatigue, leading to hypoventilation. Look for signs of T2RF and alert medical colleagues if there is cause for concern. All patients with increasing oxygen requirement or with rising (National Early Warning Score (NEWS 2) need referral to medical staff.

You can **reduce the load** on respiratory muscles by clearing airway obstruction using sputum clearance techniques (but be careful not increase fatigue). This may improve his oxygenation.

You can improve his respiratory **muscle capacity** by positioning him to enable the most efficient use of his respiratory muscles (e.g., forward lean sitting, or high side lying).

Reassurance and empathy may also help the breathless patient and may decrease WOB by reducing fear and anxiety.

If T1RF is not corrected by oxygen therapy alone, medical staff may escalate care to nasal high flow (NHF), continuous positive airway pressure (CPAP) or intubation and invasive ventilatory support.

There should be a clearly documented plan in place for if the patient does not respond to treatment. If not, you should prompt the process by approaching medical staff for clarification.

ACUTE OXYGEN THERAPY IN ADULTS

The guidance for oxygen treatment in adults in the acute setting is well evidenced and accessible on the British Thoracic Society website (O'Driscoll et al., 2017).

Oxygen is delivered according to prescription to achieve target saturations. If the patient is acutely unwell and deteriorating, or at risk of oxygen induced hypercapnic RF, they should have ABG analysis within 30 to 60 minutes of starting oxygen treatment.

OXYGEN DELIVERY DEVICES

Oxygen therapy devices can be fixed performance or variable performance devices. See Table 8.2:

Refer to local policies for advice regarding specific oxygen delivery devices.

TABLE 8.2   OXYGEN DELIVERY DEVICES

VARIABLE PERFORMANCE DEVICES, FOR EXAMPLE, SIMPLE FACE MASK OR NASAL CANNULAE	FIXED PERFORMANCE DEVICES, FOR EXAMPLE, VENTURI MASK, NASAL HIGH FLOW
Low flow devices O_2 received is dependent on minute ventilation (tidal volume × RR)	Have a high flow rate Deliver a known dose of oxygen Delivery rate exceeds minute ventilation even when the patient is tachypnoeic

When to consider humidification

Humidification is required for O_2 delivery to all artificial airways (tracheostomy) and neck breathers (laryngectomy) (National Tracheostomy Safety Project, 2013). Some patients find dry O_2 uncomfortable and humidification makes this more tolerable, potentially improving compliance. Humidification should be used for hypoxemic patients with sputum retention.

Nasal High Flow

This is increasingly being used as the first-choice treatment for T1RF. NHF delivers up to 70 L/min of heated, humidified O_2/air mix through specifically designed nasal cannula. It is well tolerated in adults with acute respiratory failure (ARF) and has shown important clinical benefit. There are a variety of proposed mechanisms by which NHF could improve clinical outcome in ARF (Table 8.3). Note that this should be prescribed in terms of both **flow** and **fraction of inspired oxygen (FiO$_2$)**.

Continuous Positive Airway Pressure

Noninvasive CPAP is the application of continuous positive airway pressure, maintained throughout the respiratory cycle, via a special face or nasal mask. Patients who require noninvasive CPAP for T1RF often require high concentrations of O_2.

The constant positive pressure delivered by CPAP improves oxygenation by increasing functional residual capacity (FRC) and improving lung compliance. These patients have widespread atelectasis because of low lung volumes.

Effects of CPAP:
- Assists alveolar recruitment
- Reduces $\dot{V}/\dot{Q}$ mismatch

TABLE 8.3	BENEFITS AND RATIONALE OF OXYGEN DELIVERY DEVICES
MECHANISM OF BENEFIT	RATIONALE
High nasal flow rates	Washes out upper airways Reduces dead space Meets inspiratory flow rates Reduces minute ventilation requirement Reduces inspiratory effort and WOB Protects the diaphragm from overuse injury
High nasal flow rates generate positive airway Pressure (2–4 cmH$_2$O)	Recruits atelectatic areas of lung Improves $\dot{V}/\dot{Q}$ matching Improves gas exchange
Heated humidified gas	Assists with sputum clearance Reduces bronchospasm Increased comfort and compliance
Fixed performance device with flow that exceeds minute ventilation, thus preventing entrainment of additional air	Increased inspired FiO$_2$ Increased alveolar oxygenation

- Improves gas exchange
- Increases arterial oxygenation
- Reduces WOB/RR
- Aids secretion mobilisation

Indications for noninvasive CPAP in T1RF include:
- Acute cardiogenic pulmonary oedema
- Postoperative patients with acute T1RF because of atelectasis
- Chest wall trauma
- Moderate to severe symptomatic obstructive sleep apnoea and hypopnoea syndrome (OSAHS) (National Institute for Health and Care Excellence, 2008)

Conditions where noninvasive CPAP is not recommended include:
- In acute asthma
- New onset T1RF where there is no history of previous lung disease, for example, diffuse pneumonia.

There is evidence that noninvasive CPAP does improve pO$_2$ in patients with diffuse pneumonia, but a trial of CPAP should be carried out in the critical care setting. Noninvasive CPAP may reduce the risk of endotracheal intubation when compared with O$_2$ delivery alone.

If treating a patient who is on noninvasive CPAP, any equipment used should be able to deliver high concentrations of O_2 to avoid desaturation. Monitor oxygenation closely throughout treatment and replace CPAP if the patient is desaturating.

Type 2 Respiratory Failure (Rochwerg et al., 2017)

Patient Story

Patient B is admitted to hospital with exacerbation of severe COPD. He is very hyperinflated. His WOB is extreme with a RR of 38. He is tripod sitting with both arms out straight and fixed. His x-ray shows hyperinflation but no consolidation or collapse. An ABG on 40% O_2 via venturi mask shows pH 7.28, pCO_2 12KPa, pO_2 7.9KPa, HCO_3 40 mmol/L, BE +4. His O_2 saturations are 88%.

Patient C has a history of advanced multiple sclerosis. She has been suffering from a chest infection for the past week, struggling to clear her secretions with a weak cough. Today, she developed sudden onset breathlessness requiring admission. On assessment, she is drowsy, opening eyes briefly to voice and has been diagnosed as having a left lower lobe collapse on chest x-ray. Her ABG on 40% O_2 via a venturi mask shows pH 7.26, pCO_2 8.4 KPa, pO_2 8.9 KPa, HCO_3 30 mmol/L, BE +3. She has been referred for respiratory physiotherapy input.

DEFINITION

T2RF occurs when:
- PaO_2 is less than 8 KPa
- $PaCO_2$ is greater than 6.5 KPa
- pH is less than 7.35
- RR is more than 24 breaths per minute

Acute T2RF occurs as a result of inadequate gas exchange and/or hypoventilation. As a result, CO_2 is retained in the body. CO_2 combines with water to make carbonic acid, so excess CO_2 leads to an acidosis and pH falling to less than 7.35. If uncorrected, the patient is likely to clinically deteriorate and be at risk of respiratory and cardiac arrest see table 8.4.

Clinical signs

The patient in T2RF will be both hypoxic and hypercapnic. See Table 7.2 (see Chapter 7, Management of work of breathing) for signs of hypoxaemia and hypercapnia.

Assessment

The priority for these patients is to reverse CO_2 retention and correct pH by optimised medical management and controlled O_2 therapy to keep oxygen saturations between 88% and 92%.

Assessment should look for reversible causes of inadequate alveolar ventilation, which could be improved by treatment. For example, improving Patient 3's gas exchange, by reversing the left lower lobe collapse caused by weak cough and sputum plugging, will improve alveolar ventilation and may reverse T2RF. Mechanical insufflation-exsufflation, assisted coughing techniques, positioning and manual techniques are all possible treatment options.

Patient B has an acute, noninfective exacerbation of COPD. He will benefit more from the pharmacological management of airway inflammation and noninvasive ventilation (NIV) than physiotherapy. Sputum retention may be an issue because narrowed and inflamed airways make it difficult to mobilise secretions. Some techniques (such as fast percussion) may worsen bronchospasm, further increasing the WOB, so caution is advised. Positioning to improve respiratory muscle capacity and reduce WOB may be helpful. Strategies to reduce dynamic hyperinflation may also be helpful, for example, pursed lip breathing, although by this stage he would benefit most from NIV.

Management

Remember, the treatment goal should be to optimise alveolar ventilation and $\dot{V}/\dot{Q}$ matching, whilst taking care not to further fatigue the respiratory muscles. If your patient is receiving NIV, ascertain how stable they are before removing NIV for treatment (e.g., do they desaturate markedly on removal of NIV?). Alternatively, controlled oxygen delivery should be delivered, as necessary, throughout treatment.

Noninvasive Ventilation

NIV is the provision of ventilatory support using a mask or similar device (interface) via the patients' upper airway. It will prevent tissue hypoxia and control respiratory acidosis, whereas other medical treatment works to reverse the precipitating cause of T2RF.

NIV can be pressure or volume controlled. Pressure controlled NIV applies an inspiratory positive airway pressure (IPAP) during inspiration and a lower expiratory positive airway pressure during

TABLE 8.4   CAUSES OF TYPE 2 RESPIRATORY FAILURE

CAUSE OF T2RF (INADEQUATE ALVEOLAR VENTILATION)	EXAMPLES
Inadequate central drive	Drug effects, e.g., opiates, brain stem lesion, head injury
Weak or fatigued respiratory muscles	Neuromuscular disease, e.g., Guillain Barré syndrome, motor neurone disease, multiple sclerosis, muscular dystrophy. High spinal injury Type 1 RF can lead to type 2 RF, as the respiratory muscles tire, leading to inadequate ventilation
Fixed thoracic cage	Kyphoscoliosis Ankylosing spondylitis Obesity hypoventilation syndrome Flail segment
Worsening of $\dot{V}/\dot{Q}$ mismatch	(Infective) COPD exacerbation
Decreased lung surface area	(Infective) exacerbation of cystic fibrosis, Bronchiectasis Pneumonia ARDS

expiration. Volume controlled devices deliver a set tidal volume to the patient. The pressure required to achieve the set volume varies from breath to breath. Volume controlled devices are particularly useful in patients who require very high pressures to achieve an adequate tidal volume, for example, chest wall disease or obesity hypoventilation. However, the vast majority of NIV is pressure controlled and tidal volumes will be augmented, but the volume will vary from breath to breath. A back up rate is also set, with associated inspiratory time, for ventilator delivered rather than spontaneous breaths.

- Increased tidal volume with each breath. If the pressure is effective, it should improve chest wall movement
- Corrects pCO_2 and pH
- Reduces RR
- Reduces WOB and breathlessness by offloading the inspiratory muscles

Indications for NIV

NIV is principally used to treat acute or chronic RF.

Contraindications

These are the few absolute contraindications to NIV: severe facial deformity, including facial fractures; facial burns; fixed upper airway obstruction; undrained pneumothorax and an inability to protect the airway.

Relative contraindications, such as excess bronchial secretions, confused and uncooperative, Glasgow coma scale less than 8, hypotension systolic BP lower than 90 mmHg, should not preclude a trial of NIV by experienced operators, in a place with a suitable level of care and enhanced observation.

Do not work beyond your competency. Use your local guidelines and do not be afraid to call for help or a second opinion. There should be a clearly documented plan in the event of treatment failure. If the patient is not responding to NIV, this may need an early referral on to Critical Care.

During assessment and treatment, it is important to check the patient is receiving adequate ventilation. Look for good chest wall excursion. Check mask fit is good, and amount of leak is not too high. Check target saturations are being achieved but not exceeded. Check patient-ventilator synchrony—does the ventilator respond with inspiratory flow to the patient making an inspiratory effort? Does it stop blowing during exhalation? (Patient-ventilator asynchrony is often because of poor mask fit and excessive leak, which is easily corrected). Ensure that the exhalation port is clear to enable CO_2 to be blown off. If the pH or pCO_2 are not responding to NIV, it may be that ventilation is not adequate—IPAP may need to be increased.

Mask comfort is very important. Discomfort resulting from an over-tight mask is a common cause of NIV failure. A full-face mask should be used for initial NIV and this should not be too tight. Pressure areas should be checked regularly and dressed to prevent pressure sores.

CONCLUSION

Physiotherapy is a key component of managing RF. Simple interventions managing sputum retention, volume loss and increased WOB can make a significant difference. Remember the patient who is not improving should be highlighted to the medical team.

References

O'Driscoll, B.R., et al., 2017. BTS guideline for oxygen use in adults in healthcare and emergency settings. Thorax 72, i1–i90.

National Tracheostomy Safety Project, 2013. www.tracheostomy.org.uk.

National Institute for Health and Care Excellence, 2008. Continuous positive airway pressure for the treatment of obstructive sleep apnoea/hypopnoea syndrome. Technology appraisal guidance Nice. org.uk/guidance/ta139.

Rochwerg, B., Brochard, L., Elliott, M.W., et al., 2017. Official ERS/ATS clinical practice guidelines: noninvasive ventilation for acute respiratory failure. ERJ 50 (2), 1602426.

RESPIRATORY PHYSIOTHERAPY TREATMENTS

Alison Draper and Paul Ritson

This alphabetically arranged list of options will assist your treatment planning. Patients respond differently, so you may consider precautions or contraindications appropriate in different circumstances for different patients. Safe and effective treatments must be your priority.

KEY MESSAGE

The scope of practice in which you are competent includes treatment techniques you have been trained to undertake. **Do not** undertake treatments outside your scope of practice. **You** are responsible for maintaining and extending this scope of practice so request regular exposure to treatment techniques you need to practise.

ABDOMINAL BREATHING

See Breathing control.

ACTIVE CYCLE OF BREATHING TECHNIQUES

Active cycle of breathing techniques ([ACBT] Fig.9.1) is a secretion clearance technique, which is a cycle of thoracic expansion exercises and forced expiration technique (FET), interspersed with breathing control. Individual components can be used separately or emphasised within the cycle, depending on the patient's symptoms. Can be used in conjunction with other treatments, including manual techniques, positioning.

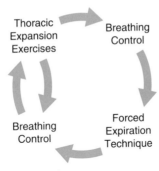

Fig. 9.1 • Active cycle of breathing techniques.

ACAPELLA®

See Oscillating positive expiratory pressure devices.

AUTOGENIC DRAINAGE

Autogenic drainage is a technique that mobilises secretions by using breathing at different lung volumes to produce high airflow in the airways (Table 9.1). Needs to be taught by physiotherapists who have had specific training in the technique.

Do not begin to teach this in an acute situation. Some patients needing emergency physiotherapy may have been taught it previously and might find it helpful.

TABLE 9.1	NOTES ON AUTOGENIC DRAINAGE	
	ADULT	CHILD/BABY
Indications	Sputum retention Taught particularly to patients with chronic lung pathology	Children as adult Babies (not applicable)
Contraindications	None	None
Precautions	None	None

BAGGING

See Manual hyperinflation.

BI-LEVEL POSITIVE AIRWAYS PRESSURE

See Noninvasive ventilation.

BOX BREATHING

- Encourage the patient to sit, well supported, in a comfortable position.
- Close their eyes, breathe through their nose for a count of 4.
- Hold their breath for a count of 4, then exhale for a count of 4.
- Repeat at least 3 times for 4 minutes, or until calm returns.

BREATHING CONTROL (BC) (DIAPHRAGMATIC BREATHING, ABDOMINAL BREATHING, RELAXED TIDAL BREATHING) (TABLE 9.2)

Relaxed breathing at tidal volume, uses minimal effort and the upper chest and shoulders should be relaxed.

- Encourage patients to breathe in through their nose (if appropriate) and breathe out gently
- A hand on the patient's abdomen encourages and monitors the rise and fall of the abdomen on inspiration and expiration. This movement will be reduced in patients with less effective diaphragmatic activity
- Use your calmest, most relaxing manner (see Relaxation techniques)
- Use positioning to support the patient's head, shoulder girdle and thorax to assist relaxation
- Give lots of encouragement, reassurance and praise
- Do not expect quick results with patients experiencing shortness of breath. They are usually reluctant and/or unable to change their breathing pattern quickly (especially those with chronic respiratory conditions)

TABLE 9.2 NOTES ON BREATHING CONTROL		
	ADULT	CHILD/BABY
Indications	Increased work of breathing Shortness of breath Altered breathing pattern Panic attacks/anxiety Hyperventilation	Children as adult. May not cooperate Babies (not applicable)
Contraindications	None	None
Precautions	Ensure patient is in a comfortable, well-supported position (see Positions of ease) Check that the patient is not actively contracting their abdominals—movement of the abdomen should be passive	As adult

- Do not insist that the patient abandons 'bad' breathing habits if they say they are helping
- Do not tell patients to 'relax' or 'slow down their breathing'—this may increase anxiety

BREATH-STACKING

Technique in which patients with neuromuscular disorders are taught to breathe in maximally, close the glottis, then breathe in maximally again, repeating this 3 to 4 times before exhaling. For patients with reduced lung volumes, this can augment inspiratory capacity and increase expiratory flow rate. Combined with expiratory techniques to aid airway clearance. Patients can be assisted with this technique using a lung volume recruitment bag, which incorporates a one-way valve.

CONTINUOUS POSITIVE AIRWAY PRESSURE

Continuous positive airway pressure ([CPAP] Table 9.3), delivered throughout both inspiration and expiration, administered to

TABLE 9.3 NOTES ON CONTINUOUS POSITIVE AIRWAY PRESSURE

	ADULT	CHILD/BABY
Indications	Increased work of breathing (WOB) or hypoxaemia caused by atelectasis, reduced FRC, flail chest, poor gas exchange across the basement membrane because of inflammation, pulmonary oedema, chronic damage	As adults
Contraindications	Undrained pneumothorax Frank haemoptysis Vomiting Facial fractures Nasal approach for neurosurgery CVS instability Raised ICP Recent upper GI surgery Active TB Lung abscess	As adults
Precautions	Increasing PaCO2 Emphysema—check CXR for large bullae Patient compliance Skin around mask can break down easily Patients with airways obstructed by a tumour—may cause air trapping Deranged platelets	As adults; children tend to dislike the sealed mask Watch the amount of CPAP given too much can cause increased WOB Start at 4 cmH2O and assess patient closely

CXR, Chest x-ray; CVS, cardiovascular system; GI, gastrointestinal; ICP, intracranial pressure; TB, tuberculosis.

a spontaneously breathing patient. Requires a high flow rate, delivered via an airtight mask, mouthpiece (with nose clip), tracheostomy tube or endotracheal (ET) tube. Can be used in treatment sessions or continuously.

- Oxygen and pressure levels should be set in liaison with medical staff. Ask for assistance from appropriate colleagues
- Patients on CPAP generally require high dependency care—check trust policy
- Other types of treatment, such as breathing exercises can be used with patients breathing with CPAP
- Benefits of CPAP are lost within minutes of removal—so it may be in the patient's best interests to stay on CPAP. However, it may be appropriate, once stabilised, to enable the patient to have short periods of time without the CPAP for personal hygiene, skin care and a drink. Monitor the patient's oxygen saturation if you remove the patient's mask for any reason, including coughing
- Humidification is recommended
- CPAP will not correct a climbing partial pressure of carbon dioxide ($PaCO_2$) in adults, but this is sometimes effective in infants under 1 year old.

CORNET (RC-CORNET®)

See Oscillating positive expiratory pressure devices.

COUGH

Reflex or voluntary mechanism for clearing airways of secretions or a foreign body (Table 9.4). An effective breath in and closure of the glottis is necessary to generate enough expiratory velocity to create an effective cough. Some patients are not able to do this. Manual support from your hands or a pillow over an incision or painful area (e.g., fractured ribs) can increase effectiveness.

- Ensure adequate pain relief before treatment.
- Allow the patient to sip a hot or cold drink intermittently during treatment if mouth is dry. For patients who are nill by mouth (NBM), let patient use mouthwash or suck an ice cube.

TABLE 9.4	NOTES ON COUGH	
	ADULT	CHILD/BABY
Indications	Prevention and treatment of sputum retention	Children as adult Babies (not applicable)
Contraindications	None	None
Precautions	Pain—ensure adequate analgesia Severe bronchospasm—avoid paroxysmal coughing Discourage unnecessary coughing in patients with significant frank haemoptysis, bleeding oesophageal varices, raised ICP (either measured or suspected) or recent cerebral bleed, major eye surgery Pertussis (whooping cough)—paroxysmal coughing can cause severe desaturation and bradycardia	As adult

ICP, Intracranial pressure.

- Ensure the patient is well-supported, leaning forward if possible, or with their knees drawn up towards their chest.
- Do not insist on repeated coughing if it is not productive.

Assisted Cough

You use manual, upwards, compression of the diaphragm given to replace the work of the abdominals to facilitate a cough in patients with spinal cord injury or neuromuscular disease (Table 9.5, Fig. 9.2).

- Two people are essential to assist coughing in patients with a spinal injury to stabilise the spine.
- Some scenarios need two people—in large patients or those with tenacious sputum.

TABLE 9.5 NOTES ON ASSISTED COUGH	ADULT	CHILD/BABY
Indications	Prevention and treatment of sputum retention	Children as adult Useful in children with degenerative neuromuscular disorders, e.g., Duchenne muscular dystrophy Babies (not applicable)
Contraindications	Pressure on abdomen should be avoided as later; direct pressure over rib fractures of chest wall injuries/ incisions should be avoided	As adult
Precautions	Immediately following surgery, especially post upper abdominal surgery, eye surgery, cardiothoracic surgery Paralytic ileus Rib fractures Raised intracranial pressure Undrained pneumothorax Osteoporosis Pain Unstable spine—an appropriate hold must be used to counter any movement	As adult

- If alone, place one hand on near side of chest and the other on the opposite side with the forearm resting on the lower ribs. As the patient coughs, push in and up with the forearm, whilst stabilising the thorax with the hands. Or both hands are placed on the lower thorax, with the elbows extended, and the physiotherapist pushes in and up with both arms.
- Take care to synchronise the assistance with the patient's attempted coughing.

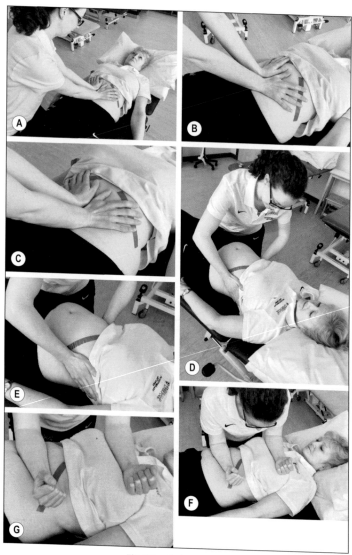

Fig. 9.2 • Assisted cough.

- Release the pressure as soon as the cough is over.
- Patients who need this help long term may have developed their own effective 'version' of this.

COUGH ASSIST DEVICE

See Manual insufflation/exsufflation device.

COUGH STIMULATION/TRACHEAL RUB

This is highly contentious—use only if it is accepted practice within your trust

DEEP BREATHING EXERCISES

See Thoracic expansion exercises.

DIAPHRAGMATIC BREATHING

See Breathing control.

FLUTTER

See Oscillatory positive expiratory pressure devices.

FORCED EXPIRATION TECHNIQUE (HUFF)

Gentle but forced breath out through an open mouth, following a breath in, which aims to move lung secretions more centrally (Table 9.6). The size of the breath in will determine the level at which sputum clearance occurs.
- Make sure the patient understands how to perform the technique effectively.

TABLE 9.6 NOTES ON FORCED EXPIRATION TECHNIQUE		
	ADULT	CHILD/BABY
Indications	Sputum retention	Children as adult Babies (not applicable)
Contraindications	None	None
Precautions	Bronchospasm	As adult

- Use analogies like 'steam up a mirror' to help your explanation.
- Encourage patients to huff from a low lung volume, that is, 'a small breath in' or 'half a breath in' to mobilise secretions in more distal airways.
- Encourage the huff from larger lung volumes, that is, after 'a deep breath in' to mobilise secretions from more proximal airways.
- Using different lung volumes may help patients with overwhelming sputum production.
- The Huff should be long enough to clear secretions – not a clearing of the throat, yet not too long (could leads to paroxysmal coughing).
- Intersperse the Huff with breathing control.
- It can be difficult to teach this technique. Try using peak flow mouthpiece or, for children, blowing games.

GRAVITY-ASSISTED DRAINAGE

See Positioning.

HIGH FLOW NASAL CANNULA

High flow nasal cannula ([HFNC]; Table 9.7) is a delivery of gas up to 70 litres per minute via nasal cannula to adults, infants and children. To make this tolerable, it requires heating and humidification. The flow and fraction of inspired oxygen (FiO_2) need to be prescribed.

TABLE 9.7	HIGH FLOW NASAL CANNULA (OPTIFLOW/VAPOTHERM/AIRVO)	
	ADULT	CHILD/BABY
Indications	Increased work of breathing High oxygen requirement Poor tolerance of face mask Patients who may benefit from humidity/ assistance clearing secretions	As adult
Contraindications	Maxillofacial trauma Complete nasal obstruction Basal skull fracture Undrained pneumothorax	As adult
Precautions	Ensure flow not too high for patient Should not have forced expiration if flow appropriate	As adult Start at flow of 2 litres per kilo body weight and titrate accordingly

HUFF

See Forced expiration technique.

HUMIDIFICATION

Inhaled water vapour or aerosol administered by mask (Table 9.8).
- Many different types of equipment are available, familiarise yourself with what your trust uses.
- The water vapour may be cold or heated.
- Wide diameter tubing (21 mm) and a mask are essential for effective delivery.

TABLE 9.8 NOTES ON HUMIDIFICATION

	ADULT	CHILD/BABY
Indications	Sputum retention, particularly thick sticky secretions, difficulty expectorating, dry mouth Patients needing continuous oxygen (dry gas) Patients breathing via a tracheostomy/ endotracheal tube (the natural warming mechanism of the nasal passages is bypassed)	As adult
Contraindications	None	None
Precautions	Patients prone to bronchospasm may react to nebulised water. Use saline if required— this will reduce the lifespan of the humidification unit as the saline will crystallise Airway/facial burns if heated humidification is unmonitored (all equipment should have temperature gauges and alarms) Can exacerbate fluid overload in cardiac conditions	Given via head box in infants and mask in children

- Give humidification time to be effective. If starting humidification as part of your treatment, allow 10 to 15 minutes before (re)commencing sputum clearance techniques.
- Cold air blowing onto heated humidification tubing, from fans or open windows, will cause water to collect in the tubing—this should be emptied regularly.

- Humidification units should not be left switched off and then re-used as they become an infection hazard.
- An alternative is to consider regular prescribed saline nebulisers (usually 5 mL of 0.9% saline) and appropriate systemic hydration. Only use humidification if these are not effective.

HYPERTONIC SALINE

See Nebulised hypertonic saline or mucolytics.

INCENTIVE SPIROMETER

Incentive spirometer is a device which gives visual feedback on the performance of a slow deep breath in (Table 9.9). There is little evidence in the literature for its use.
- Patients need to be able to remember how to use the device when you are not there, so give clear instructions.
- Ask the patient to adopt a position which facilitates deep breathing (see Positioning to increase volume).
- Be aware that patients quickly learn to cheat—ensure what you are seeing is being produced by a slow deep breath in.
- Unhelpful if patients are breathless.
- Do not use with patients requiring a high concentration of oxygen by mask.

TABLE 9.9 NOTES ON INCENTIVE SPIROMETER		
	ADULT	CHILD/BABY
Indications	Volume loss. May be useful for patients who have difficulty with understanding the concept of thoracic expansion exercises	Children as adult. Limited to use by older children Babies (not applicable)
Contraindications	None	None
Precautions	None	None

INDUCED SPUTUM

See Nebulised hypertonic saline or mucolytics.

INSPIRATORY MUSCLE TRAINING

Inspiratory muscle training (IMT) is a device providing resistance to inspiration, increasing load and strengthening inspiratory muscles. A regime related to the patient's 1-rep-max (1RM) can be prescribed. This is not suitable in acutely unwell patients. Consider it when patients are severely deconditioned with respiratory muscle weakness, such as those recovering from prolonged mechanical ventilation.

INTERMITTENT POSITIVE PRESSURE BREATHING

Intermittent positive pressure breathing (IPPB) is an intermittent treatment, which delivers positive pressure on inspiration only, to increase lung expansion and support the action of the respiratory muscles (Table 9.10). Breaths are delivered by mouthpiece or face mask and triggered by the patient's inspiratory effort. The old IPPB "BIRD" machines are being phased out. Manual insufflation/exsufflation devices can provide a similar effect to IPPB. Troubleshooting is the same.

Helpful Hints

- Position the patient with the affected lung uppermost or in a position to facilitate deep breathing (see Positioning to increase volume).
- Adult settings for IPPB where numbered dials are present:
  - Sensitivity—keep low, unless the machine appears to be triggering too easily
  - Flow rate—start at mid range. If the patient is very breathless, start with a high flow and be prepared to adjust it, until the breath in is fast enough for the patient
  - Pressure—start at 10 cmH$_2$O and aim to increase depending on the response of the patient during the treatment
- DO NOT use in children if they are uncompliant or under 5 years of age. Suggest starting pressures: 10 cmH$_2$O then increase to 20 to 25 cmH$_2$O maximum.

TABLE 9.10	NOTES ON INTERMITTENT POSITIVE PRESSURE BREATHING	
	ADULT	CHILD/BABY
Indications	Increased WOB, sputum retention, poor tidal volume particularly in weak or tired patients	As adult Children older than 6 years of age seem to be able to comply
Contraindications	Undrained pneumothorax Frank haemoptysis Vomiting blood (haematemesis) Facial fractures, nasal approach for neurosurgery CVS instability Raised ICP Recent lung/upper GI surgery Active TB Lung abscess	As adult
Precautions	Emphysema—check CXR for bullae Patients with airways obstructed by a tumour—may cause air trapping Deranged platelets	As adult

CXR, Chest x-ray; CVS, cardiovascular system; GI, gastrointestinal; ICP, intracranial pressure; TB, tuberculosis, WOB, work of breathing.

- Try to ensure that after triggering the machine, the rest of the inspiratory phase is passive; the patient needs to let the machine to do the work during inspiration.
- Ensure the set pressure is achieved on full inspiration. If the pressure swings above the set level, it suggests the patient is blowing into the machine—the machine cuts out early and set pressures are not transmitted to the lungs.
- Use 0.9% saline if the machine has a nebuliser.
- An effective seal is essential. This can be achieved by a tight seal with the face mask (make sure that the head is supported so you

can hold the mask securely in place) or a mouthpiece with the nose pinched or a nose clip.

- Use for short periods of time, for example, 10 minutes every hour. Do not to give the patient more than four to eight breaths in a row. If nursing staff are to assist with this therapy ensure they are familiar with the equipment, the risk of pneumothorax, and do not change the settings.
- Do not allow the patient to use the machine unsupervised, unless you are confident they can use it effectively.
- If things are going wrong and you lose confidence with the equipment, take the machine away, use a clean circuit, and try the machine on yourself to sort out the problems. Go back to the patient and start again.

LATERAL COSTAL BREATHING

See Thoracic expansion exercises.

LUNG VOLUME RECRUITMENT BAG

See Breath stacking.

MANUAL HYPERINFLATION

Deep breaths delivered manually to a mechanically ventilated patient by means of a rebreathing bag, commonly referred to as *bagging or MHI* (Table 9.11). Slow deep inspiration recruits collateral ventilation, expands areas of atelectasis and improves arterial blood gases (ABGs). An inspiratory hold at full inspiration will further promote lung expansion (not helpful in patients prone to air trapping, e.g., emphysema). A fast-expiratory release mimics the FET and may stimulate coughing. It is possible to maintain positive end expiratory pressure (PEEP) either, held by hand or by means of a PEEP valve.

- Some critical care units have a policy of using ventilator-delivered inspiratory holds and sighs or ventilator hyperinflation (VHI) instead of MHI. Check your trust policy before undertaking.
- Use a 2-L bag for adults, a 500-mL open-ended bag for babies, 1-L bag for children.

TABLE 9.11   NOTES ON MANUAL HYPERINFLATION

	ADULT	CHILD/BABY
Indications	Intubated patients with atelectasis or sputum retention hypoxia	As adults
Contraindications	Undrained pneumothorax CVS instability/arrhythmias Systolic BP <80 mmHg Severe bronchospasm Peak airway pressure >40 cmH_2O when mechanically ventilated High PEEP requirement >15 cmH_2O Unexplained haemoptysis Raised ICP above the set limits	As adults Systolic BP <55 mmHg (infants) or <75 mmHg (children >2 years)
Precautions	Use a manometer to monitor peak pressures if available. Do not exceed 40 cmH_2O pressure PEEP >10 cmH_2O—only bag if essential. Use PEEP valve while bagging if patient is PEEP dependent Drained pneumothorax Recent lung surgery (within last 14 days) Arrhythmias or unstable BP On 100% O_2 (FiO_2 1)— disconnection from the ventilator may cause sudden desaturation Watch the monitor for changes in HR or BP Reduced respiratory drive—an air/oxygen mix may be preferable Raised ICP within the set limits	High-frequency oscillation—leave on ventilator as much as possible Unstable BP Monitor peak volume and pressure as pneumothorax easily happens Raised ICP within the set limits

BP, Blood pressure; *CVS,* cardiovascular system; *ICP,* intracranial pressure; *HR,* heart rate; *FIO₂,* fraction of inspired oxygen; *PEEP,* positive end expiratory pressure.

- Do not bag a child if you are inexperienced with this age group. Paediatric bags have an open-end valve and this technique needs practise to achieve safe, effective bagging.
- Use a manometer in the circuit. For children, give approximately 10% above ventilator setting – positive inspiratory pressure (PIP)/PEEP.
- If you are not confident with the technique, ask the nurse to assist you by bagging, while you undertake physiotherapy techniques; this is perfectly appropriate.
- If possible, position the patient with the area of atelectasis or sputum retention uppermost. Side lying is often the most appropriate position, but not always possible to achieve.
- Watch the patient's chest to assess lung expansion.
- Coordinate the procedure with the patient's own breathing if they can cooperate.
- Stop when secretions are heard
- Aim to mimic ACBT with no more than three or four hyperinflations in succession; do not give more than eight.
- Do not continue if patient becomes distressed, systolic blood pressure drops below 80 mmHg (55 mmHg in infants and 75 mmHg in children over 2 years of age), arrhythmias develop or intracranial pressure (ICP) increases beyond limits for that patient set by neurosurgeon or intensivist.

MANUAL INSUFFLATION/EXSUFFLATION (COUGH ASSIST, CLEARWAY)

Device to assists cough effort by means of a positive pressure breath, followed by a rapid switch to negative pressure (Table 9.12). Most effective in patients with an ineffective cough because of neuromuscular weakness. However, its use is increasing with other groups of patients. Can be adapted for use as IPPB (see IPPB).

- Fear, pain and poor technique will lead to poor synchrony with the machine and an ineffective treatment.
- A tight seal is essential—use a face mask, mouthpiece with nose clip, or catheter mount for tracheostomy or intubated patients; coughing is easier with a face mask.
- Either you need to synchronise the breath in and breath out with the patient, or the automatic mode can be used, establish which the patient finds most comfortable.

TABLE 9.12	NOTES ON MANUAL INSUFFLATION/EXSUFFLATION (COUGH ASSIST/CLEARWAY)	
	ADULT	CHILD/BABY
Indications	Prevention and treatment of sputum retention	Children as adult Babies (not applicable)
Contraindications	Undrained pneumothorax	As adult
Precautions	Oxygen dependency; entrain oxygen into the breathing circuit Do not instigate use in the on-call setting if you are not fully trained and confident Bronchospasm	As adult

BP, Blood pressure; *CVS*, cardiovascular system.

- Instruct the patient to cough when the breath out starts, they may also need a few inspiratory breaths after coughing to recover.
- Start with a low inspiratory pressure, for example, 10 cmH$_2$O, and gradually increase the pressure to achieve a deep breath with the patient. If on noninvasive ventilation (NIV), start at the level set on the ventilator; initially keep inspiratory and expiratory pressures equal. Then increase expiratory pressure if the patient needs a stronger 'cough'. A maximum inspiratory pressure of 40 cmH$_2$O is recommended, but check your trust policy.
- You can combine this with manual techniques and an assisted cough.

MANUAL TECHNIQUES

See Percussion, shaking and vibrations

MOBILISATION

In the acute situation, patients may not be well enough to mobilise. It may be necessary to help the patient move to get them into a more appropriate position for treatment (Table 9.13). Any activity requiring physical effort can induce spontaneous deep breathing and associated

TABLE 9.13	NOTES ON MOBILISATION	
	ADULT	CHILD/BABY
Indications	Sputum retention Volume loss Limited to previously mobile patients	Children as adult A toddler may need assistance to mobilise Babies—ensure that the baby is able to roll and move around the cot—THIS IS STILL MOBILISING THE PATIENT!
Contraindications	CVS instability Low BP, serious arrhythmia	As adult
Precautions	Drips, drains and catheters Ensure pain controlled Follow local protocols for patients with epidural analgesia or postorthopaedic, plastic and vascular surgery	As adult

BP, Blood pressure; *CVS*, cardiovascular system.

increases in expiratory flow rates can help loosen secretions. It can also provoke coughing and help increase respiratory muscle strength.
- Ensure you have sufficient help before attempting to get a patient out of bed.
- Work with the patient enabling them to assist in the manoeuvre as much as possible.
- A child in pain will be reluctant to mobilise; ensure adequate analgesia and use your powers of persuasion!

NEBULISED HYPERTONIC SALINE OR MUCOLYTICS

Nebulised hypertonic saline (≤7% sodium chloride solution) hydrates the mucociliary escalator potentially reducing sputum viscosity and assisting sputum clearance in patients with chronic airways disease Table 9.14). Mucolytics can be nebulised (e.g., N acetyl cysteine, DNAse) or oral (e.g., Carbocisteine);both breakdown sputum, making it less thick and easier to expectorate. All need prescription.

TABLE 9.14   NOTES ON NEBULISED HYPERTONIC SALINE

	ADULT	CHILD/BABY
Indications	Sputum retention	
Contraindications	Closely monitor patients with haemoptysis	As adult
Precautions	May cause bronchospasm Hypertonic saline must not be mixed with any other drugs Avoid giving other inhaled medication immediately beforehand	As adult

Nebulised hypertonic saline can be used to facilitate production of sputum sample for analysis when not possible by other methods of airway clearance (sputum induction/induced sputum). Check your trust policy and get appropriate training.

NEUROPHYSIOLOGIC FACILITATION OF RESPIRATION

The use of proprioceptive and tactile stimuli to produce a reflex respiratory response in unconscious patients, to improve ventilatory activity.

NONINVASIVE VENTILATION

Noninvasive ventilation (Table 9.15) provides ventilator support via a tight-fitting interface (mouth piece, nasal pillows, face or nasal mask). The aim of the treatment is to increase the minute volume (tidal volume × respiratory rate [RR]) and thus either stabilise or reduce $PaCO_2$. In modern ventilators, this is achieved by the application of varying pressures throughout the respiratory cycle. The inspiratory positive airway pressure is higher than the expiratory positive airway pressure. The pressure difference drives the ventilation. In some older machines, the delivered tidal volume was the setting changed. There are some modern ventilators which combine the two systems to guarantee a set level of support.

TABLE 9.15 NOTES ON NONINVASIVE VENTILATION

	ADULT	CHILD/BABY
Indications	Increased WOB causing ventilatory failure, i.e., increased CO_2, fatigue, neuromuscular disorders	As adult
Contraindications	Undrained pneumothorax Frank haemoptysis Vomiting blood (haematemesis) Facial fractures CVS instability Raised ICP Recent upper GI surgery Active TB Lung abscess	As adults
Precautions	Emphysema—check CXR for bullae Patient compliance Skin around mask can easily break down Patients with airways obstructed by a tumour – may cause air trapping	As adults Children may dislike the sealed mask

CXR, Chest x-ray; CVS, cardiovascular system; GI, gastrointestinal; ICP, intracranial pressure; TB, tuberculosis, WOB, work of breathing.

Helpful Hints

- The decision to use NIV and the settings chosen must always be made with the multidisciplinary team.
- Introduce the treatment to the patient slowly and ensure that the mask is comfortable.
- Allow the patient to practise taking some breaths, while they hold the mask in place, without fastening the straps.
- Patient must be able to keep the mouth closed with a nasal mask.
- Listen to the patient's concerns, some patients are less suited to NIV and they should be individually assessed.
- NIV should be used in intensive care unit/high dependency units or specialist respiratory care environments for the acutely unwell patient—check your trust policy.

OSCILLATING POSITIVE EXPIRATORY DEVICES

- Acapella® (Fig. 9.3A)
- AerobiKA (Fig. 9.3B)
- Turboforte®/PARI O-PEP/Flutter® (Fig. 9.3C)
- RC-Cornet® (Fig. 9.3D)
- Bubble PEP (Fig. 9.3E)

Devices which can be used alone or with other techniques to treat retained secretions. Exhaling through the device results in positive expiratory pressure (PEP) and vibration within the airways to loosen

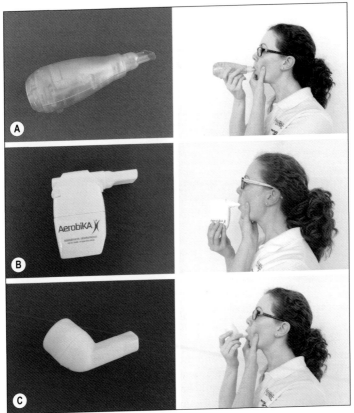

Fig. 9.3 • Oscillatory positive expiratory pressure devices (A) Acapella. (B) AerobiKA. (C) Flutter.

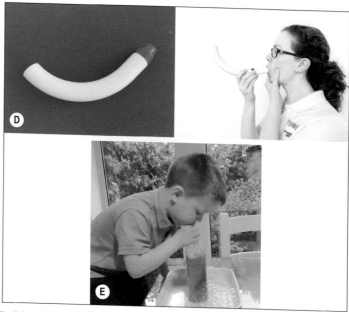

Fig. 9.3, cont'd • (D) RC-Cornet. (E) Bubble PEP.

TABLE 9.16	NOTES ON OSCILLATING POSITIVE EXPIRATORY PRESSURE DEVICES	
	ADULT	CHILD/BABY
Indications	Sputum retention	Children as adult Babies (not applicable)
Precautions	None	Younger children may dislike sealed mask
Contraindications	None	None

secretions (Table 9.16). Consider using in an acute situation if you are familiar with these devices and they are regularly used in your trust.
- Not a first-line emergency treatment but patients can continue to use the device if they already have one and feel it is helpful.
- The patient holds the device themselves, make sure they maintain an airtight seal.

- Treatment time is 5 to 15 minutes and intersperse with FET.
- Adjust the angle of the Turboforte®/PARI O-PEP/Flutter® to achieve maximal oscillation.

OVERPRESSURE

Manual pressure applied to the ribcage at the end of the breath out and quickly released to stimulate inspiration. Consider carefully before using in patients with chest trauma/postsurgery and fragile ribs, for example, osteoporosis.

OXYGEN THERAPY

Delivering oxygen at a higher concentration than in room air between 24% and 100%. Give the minimum dose necessary to have the effect you want, because oxygen is toxic if given (unnecessarily) in high concentrations over a prolonged period (Table 9.17).

TABLE 9.17 NOTES ON OXYGEN THERAPY		
	ADULT	CHILD/BABY
Indications	Hypoxaemia Before and after suction	As adult
Contraindications	None	Duct-dependent cardiac lesions – follow local protocols
Precautions	Hypercapnic COPD patients who may be dependent on hypoxaemia for respiratory drive – use ABGs to assess	Remember humidification via mask or HFNC if >2 L/min

ABGs, Arterial blood gases; *COPD*, chronic obstructive pulmonary disease; *HFNC*, high flow nasal cannula.

Should be prescribed in adults with a target saturation. Give as necessary, without prescription, in paediatrics (unless there is an underlying duct-dependent cardiac lesion). Changes to dose (other than when preoxygenating for suction) must be discussed with the medical team.

- Ensure adequate humidification is provided with high concentrations and continuous use.
- All tracheostomy and laryngectomy patients requiring oxygen, should have humidification.

PERCUSSION

Rhythmic clapping on the patient's chest with cupped hands to assist secretion clearance (Table 9.18).

- For adults and older children use in conjunction with thoracic expansion exercises.
- Cushion the area with a folded towel and use a good technique—patient comfort is important.

TABLE 9.18 NOTES ON PERCUSSION		
	ADULT	CHILD/BABY
Indications	Sputum retention	As adult
Contraindications	Directly over rib fracture Directly over a surgical incision or graft Frank haemoptysis Severe osteoporosis Hypoxia—percussion can exacerbate hypoxia, especially in infants	As adult
Precautions	Profound hypoxaemia Bronchospasm, pain Osteoporosis, bony metastases Near chest drains	Baby—make sure head is supported

TABLE 9.19 NOTES ON GRAVITY ASSISTED DRAINAGE

	ADULT	CHILD/BABY
Indications	Sputum retention, particularly if localised to one lung segment or lobe	As adult
Contraindications to head-down position	Hypertension Severe dyspnoea Recent surgery Severe haemoptysis Nose bleeds Advanced pregnancy Hiatus hernia Cardiac failure Cerebral oedema Aortic aneurysm Head or neck trauma/surgery Mechanical ventilation	As adult
Precautions	Diaphragmatic paralysis/weakness	Head-down position can cause reflux, vomiting and aspiration, and splints the diaphragm reducing respiratory effectiveness

POSITIONING: GRAVITY-ASSISTED DRAINAGE (POSTURAL DRAINAGE)

Positions which use gravity to drain retained secretions (Tables 9.19 and 9.20).

Helpful Hints

- Do not use head-down tilt immediately after meals/feed or if there are any contraindications.
- Position should be maintained for approximately 10 minutes.
- Can be modified to side lying (affected lung uppermost), with or without head-down tilt for generalised secretions.
- Drain worst affected area first.
- Most hospital beds have a catch at the bottom of the bed or an electric switch to tip the bed

TABLE 9.20   GRAVITY-ASSISTED DRAINAGE POSITIONS

LOBE	SEGMENT	POSITION
Upper lobe	Apical bronchus Right posterior bronchus Left posterior bronchus Anterior bronchus	Sitting upright Lying on the left side horizontally turned 45 degrees on to the face, resting against a pillow, with another supporting the head Lying on the right side turned 45 degrees on to the face, with three pillows arranged to lift the shoulders 30 cm from the horizontal Lying supine with the knees flexed
Lingula	Superior and inferior bronchus	Lying supine with the body a quarter turned to the right maintained by a pillow under the left side from shoulder to hip. The chest is tilted downwards to an angle of 15 degrees
Middle lobe	Lateral bronchus Medial bronchus	Lying supine with the body a quarter turned to the left maintained by a pillow under the right side from shoulder to hip. The chest is tilted downwards to an angle of 15 degrees
Lower lobe	Apical basal bronchus Anterior basal bronchus Medial basal bronchus Lateral basal bronchus Posterior basal bronchus	Lying prone with a pillow under the abdomen Lying supine with the knees flexed and the chest tilted downwards to an angle of 20 degrees Lying on the right side with the chest tilted downwards to an angle of 20 degrees Lying on the left side with the chest tilted downwards to an angle of 20 degrees Lying prone with a pillow under the hips and the chest tilted downwards to an angle of 20 degrees

- Postural drainage may result in a V/Q mismatch especially in children. Discuss this with the medical team and adapt the position or temporarily increase the oxygen.

POSITIONING TO INCREASE LUNG VOLUME

Positioning of spontaneously breathing patients to facilitate maximal inspiration and improve functional residual capacity ([FRC], Table 9.21).

TABLE 9.21	NOTES ON POSITIONING TO INCREASE LUNG VOLUME	
	ADULT	CHILD/BABY
Indications	Volume loss, i.e., poor expansion because of pain, fear of pain, immobility	As adult
Contraindications	Cardiovascular system instability Unstable spinal fracture Unstable head injury	As adult
Precautions	Proceed slowly if standing the patient for the first time after a period of bed rest	As adult

Use the most upright position the patient can tolerate, for example, standing, high sitting; otherwise side lying is acceptable.
• Get as much help as necessary to move the patient safely.

POSITIONING: POSITIONS OF EASE

Well-supported, positioning of spontaneously breathing patients to encourages relaxation of the upper chest and shoulders and 'free' the diaphragm (Fig. 9.4A–F and Table 9.22).

POSITIONING: PRONE

Mechanically ventilated patients, with profound hypoxic, may be nursed in the prone position to aid recruitment of lung tissue and chest physiotherapy is possible if appropriate. Most patients nursed prone do not have sputum retention but require high levels of PEEP and oxygen so may not benefit from physiotherapy. Be aware of the need to protect neural and soft tissues in this position. Fig. 9.5A shows the recommended upper limb position, but this may need to be modified (as shown in Fig. 9.5B and C).

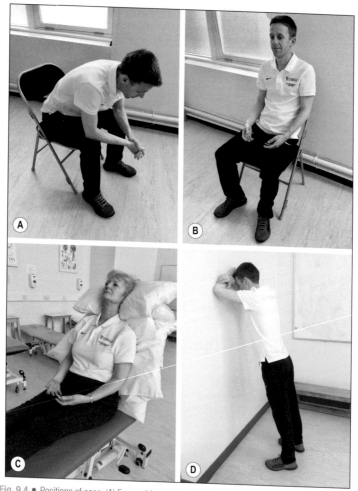

Fig. 9.4 • Positions of ease. (A) Forward-lean sitting. (B) Relaxed sitting. (C) Half lying (D) Forward-lean standing.

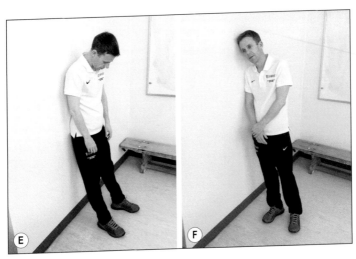

Fig. 9.4, cont'd • (E and F) Relaxed standing.

TABLE 9.22	NOTES ON POSITIONS OF EASE	
	ADULT	CHILD/BABY
Indications	Increased work of breathing Shortness of breath at rest and on exercise Anxiety/panic attacks Hyperventilation	Children as adult Babies see Fig. 9.5
Contraindications	None	None
Precautions	None	None

This position is used commonly in children because of its positive effect on gas exchange. If you use this position, make sure they are carefully monitored (i.e., heart rate [HR], blood pressure [BP], oxygen saturation [SpO$_2$], RR) because of the link to sudden infant death syndrome.

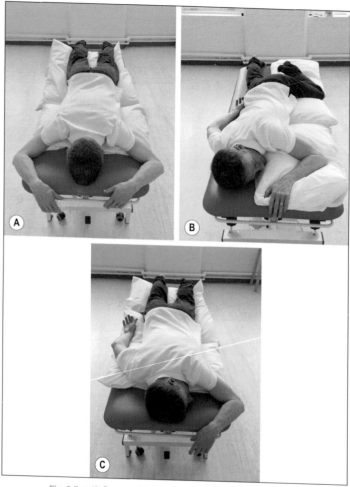

Fig. 9.5 • (A) Prone position and (B and C) suggested modifications.

TABLE 9.23	NOTES ON POSITIONING TO MATCH VENTILATION/ PERFUSION	
	ADULT	CHILD/BABY
Indications	Hypoxaemia	As adult
Contraindications	Cardiovascular system instability Unstable spinal fracture Unstable head injury	As adult
Precautions	Proceed slowly if standing the patient for the first time after a period of bed rest	As adult
Ventilated	Lung with pathology down	Lung with pathology up (baby and small child)
Nonventilated	Lung with pathology up	Lung with pathology down (baby and small child)

POSITIONING: VENTILATION/PERFUSION MATCHING

Positioning which maximises ventilation perfusion matching in patients with unilateral lung pathology (Table 9.23).

- Get as much help as necessary to safely move the patient.
- Ensure you understand the principles of ventilation and perfusion before deciding how to position the patient—dependent parts of lung are preferentially ventilated and perfused in spontaneously breathing adults.
- Babies, small children and mechanically ventilated adults preferentially ventilate nondependent lung areas but perfuse dependent regions and it is difficult to match ventilation and perfusion in these patients.

POSITIVE EXPIRATORY PRESSURE DEVICES (TABLE 9.24)

These can be used alone or in conjunction with other techniques to treat retained secretions (Table 9.24). Exhaling through a mask or

TABLE 9.24 NOTES ON POSITIVE EXPIRATORY PRESSURE DEVICES

	ADULT	CHILD/BABY
Indications	Sputum retention	Children as adult Babies (not applicable)
Precautions	None	Younger children may dislike sealed mask
Contraindications	None	None

mouthpiece results in PEP in the airways, which loosens secretions. Consider using in an acute setting if you are familiar with these and they are used in your workplace.

- Not an emergency treatment, but patients can continue to use them if they feel it helps.
- The patient should hold the device themselves and ensure an airtight seal.
- Frequency and duration of treatment depends on sputum volumes, dyspnoea and fatigue.
- Use with frequent FET.
- Some devices may incorporate the use of a nebulizer.
- With a PEP mask and manometer, the pressure should be between 10 and 20 cmH$_2$O during mid-expiration.
- A mouthpiece with nose clip can be used instead of a mask.

POSTURAL DRAINAGE

See Positioning.

RELAXATION TECHNIQUES

These help patients reduce unhelpful muscle tension and anxiety, which contributes to increased work of breathing (Table 9.25). You need to use an appropriate voice, calm manner. Advise on positioning, breathing and specific relaxation techniques, such as 'visualisation', or 'contract/relax'

TABLE 9.25	NOTES ON RELAXATION TECHNIQUES	
	ADULT	CHILD/BABY
Indications	Increased WOB SOB at rest and on exercise Altered breathing pattern Panic attacks, anxiety Hyperventilation	Children as adult Babies (not applicable)
Precautions	None	None
Contraindications	None	None

SOB, Shortness of breath; WOB, work of breathing.

- Ensure you are relaxed when trying to reduce tension in your patient!
- Position the patient in a comfortable well supported position—forward-lean sitting or high side lying are useful if the patient is breathless (see positions of ease).
- Incorporate elements of relaxation into the management of the breathing problem.
- Be aware that a noisy bustling ward is not ideal for relaxation.

RELAXED TIDAL BREATHING

See Breathing control.

RIB SPRINGING

Used in the paralysed patient, manual compression of the chest wall, continued throughout expiration with the application of overpressure at the end of the breath out. A quick release encourages inspiration. Care is needed with the amount of compression applied because the patient is unable to report pain. Contraindicated for babies and all patients with fragile ribs/vertebrae (e.g., osteoporosis).

SALINE NEBULISER

See Humidification.

TABLE 9.26	NOTES ON SHAKING	
	ADULT	CHILD/BABY
Indications	Sputum retention	Sputum retention
Contraindications	Directly over rib fracture or surgical incision	Premature infants— causes brain injury, DO NOT USE
Precautions	Long-term oral steroids/ osteoporosis, bony metastases Near chest drains Severe bronchospasm Rib fractures	Baby—make sure head is supported

SHAKING

Coarse oscillations produced by the therapist's hands compressing and releasing the chest wall. Performed during thoracic expansion exercises, only on exhalation, after a deep breath in (Table 9.26).
* This should not be uncomfortable, ask the patient

SPUTUM INDUCTION/INDUCED SPUTUM

See Nebulised hypertonic saline or mucolytics.

SUCTION

Endotracheal/tracheostomy suction
Removal of secretions from the upper airways, using a suction catheter, in patients who are intubated or have a tracheostomy (Table 9.27).
* Pre-/postoxygenate, before and after suction, either by manual hyperinflation or increasing the baseline FiO_2 on the ventilator according to the trust policy.
* Use each catheter once unless closed system suction is used.
* Discontinue if arrhythmias develop, or HR/BP drops.
* Explain the procedure to the patient with lots of reassurance.

TABLE 9.27 NOTES ON ENDOTRACHEAL SUCTION

	ADULT	CHILD/BABY
Indications	Sputum retention in intubated patients Sputum retention may be indicated by high peak airway pressures with volume-controlled ventilation or decreased tidal volume with pressure-controlled ventilation, auscultation, hypoxaemia or reduced SpO_2 Visible/audible secretions not effectively removed with a cough and causing respiratory distress Poor cough caused by neurologic pathology, pain inhibition, or inhibition by drugs Aspiration Reduced tidal volumes in ventilated patients Increased peak pressures in ventilated patients	Sputum retention indicated by increased work of breathing in association with other signs: Decreased SpO_2/hypoxia Deteriorating blood gases in association with other indications Increased HR Auscultation in association with other indications
Contraindications	None if indicated	As adult
Precautions	Low SpO_2 Dependency on high O_2 High ventilatory requirements (closed circuit catheters will reduce need to disconnect patient from ventilator) Severe CVS instability Anticoagulated patients or those with clotting disorders Severe bronchospasm Recent lung oesophageal surgery	As adult

CVS, cardiovascular system; *HR*, heart rate, SpO_2, oxygen saturation.

Suction catheter size guide:
- Child—internal diameter of ET or tracheostomy tube in millimetres multiplied by 2, for example, tube size 3.5 mm × 2 = size 7 (French gauge) suction catheter.
- Adult internal diameter of ET or tracheostomy tube in millimetres, multiply by 3 then divide by 2. For example, tube size 8 × 3 / 2 = size 12.

Nasopharyngeal/Pharyngeal Suction

Removal of secretions from the upper airways by means of a suction catheter introduced via the nose or mouth (Table 9.28). In general,

TABLE 9.28   NOTES ON NASOPHARYNGEAL SUCTION

	ADULT	CHILD/BABY
Indications	Retained secretions/aspiration in the upper airways of patients who are unable to cough or have reduced cough caused by fatigue, neurologic pathology, pain inhibition, or inhibition by drugs	Visible/audible secretions not effectively removed with a cough and causing respiratory distress Poor cough caused by neurologic pathology, pain inhibition, or inhibition by drugs Aspiration
Contraindications	Stridor Skull fractures Craniofacial surgery/injury	As adult Haemangioma
Precautions	High malignancy, high oesophageal varices Anticoagulated patients or those with clotting disorders Severe CVS instability Severe bronchospasm Recent pneumonectomy or oesophagectomy – liaise with surgeons	As adult

CVS, Cardiovascular system.

in patients who are unconscious/semiconscious or neurologically
impaired and unable to clear secretions effectively.

- Use an airway for oral suction or frequent nasal suctioning.
- Preoxygenate the patient.
- Position the patient in side lying in case they vomit.
- Use a 'clean' technique.
- Do not use if the patient would require physical restraint to carry
  out the procedure.
- Do not suction patients to remove pulmonary oedema as the oede-
  ma will be replaced.
- Remember to give lots of reassurance.
- Some units will insert a mini-tracheostomy (a thin blue tube)
  into the trachea if repeated suction is needed. This procedure
  is associated with as much risk as formal tracheostomy insertion. Mini-tracheostomy is not used in the majority of paediatric
  units.
- Try to avoid using oropharyngeal suction in babies as this increases
  the risk of vomiting and aspiration.

THORACIC EXPANSION (DEEP BREATHING EXERCISES, LATERAL COSTAL BREATHING)

Maximal breath in followed by relaxed expiration (Table 9.29). Can be
used in conjunction with manual techniques (e.g., percussion, vibrations or shaking) or with inspiratory hold and/or sniff to increase the
depth of the breath and improve collateral ventilation.

- Inspiratory hold: breath-hold for a few seconds at the end of a deep
  breath in.
- Sniff: sniff in through the nose at the end of a deep breath in.
- Use your hands to give firm support on the lateral aspects of the patient's ribcage (above the level of rib 8) to monitor the performance
  and give sensory input.
- Use your voice to give lots of encouragement.
- Avoid placing your hands directly over an incision or painful area of
  the chest.
- Do not ask the patient to perform more than three or four deep
  breaths at a time (they may become light-headed).

TABLE 9.29 NOTES ON THORACIC EXPANSION EXERCISES		
	ADULT	CHILD/BABY
Indications	Poor expansion because of lung collapse Sputum retention or atelectasis, pain, fear of pain or immobility	Children as adult Babies (not applicable)
Contraindications	None	None
Precautions	Ensure that the patient has received adequate analgesia, if appropriate, before commencing treatment Ensure that the patient is in a suitable position (see Positioning to increase volume)	As adult

- Patients who are breathless will not be able to perform consecutive thoracic expansion exercises (TEEs).
- Intersperse TEEs with breathing control.

VENTILATOR HYPERINFLATION

See Manual hyperinflation.

VIBRATIONS

Fine oscillations applied to the chest wall by the therapist's hands or fingertips (in babies). Performed during thoracic expansion exercises, on exhalation (Table 9.30).
- Use firm contact and direct the force inwards towards the centre of the chest.
- Perform on expiration phase after a deep breath in.

TABLE 9.30 NOTES ON VIBRATIONS		
	ADULT	CHILD/BABY
Indications	Sputum retention	Sputum retention
Contraindications	Directly over rib fracture or surgical incision Severe bronchospasm	Premature infants— may cause brain injury if head is unsupported
Precautions	Long-term oral steroids/ osteoporosis Near chest drains Rib fractures	Make sure head is supported

Further Reading

Hough, A., 2017. Hough's Cardiorespiratory Care, fifth ed. Elsevier, Edinburgh.

Main, E., Denehy, L., 2016. Cardiorespiratory Physiother, fifth ed. Elsevier, Edinburgh.

CHAPTER 10

WORKING ON SURGICAL WARDS

Valerie Ball and Jayne Anderson

On the surgical ward, your role is to minimise the impact of postoperative pulmonary complications (PPC), encourage early mobility (alongside other members of the multidisciplinary team) and facilitate the most appropriate discharge destination, based on functional ability. A PPC is an infection, respiratory failure, pleural effusion, atelectasis, pneumothorax, bronchospasm, aspiration pneumonitis, pneumonia, adult respiratory distress syndrome (ARDS), tracheobronchitis, pulmonary oedema or exacerbation of preexisting chronic chest conditions (Miskovic and Lumb, 2017). The incidence of PPCs is declining with improvements in surgical management including, minimally invasive laparoscopic procedures, enhanced recovery after surgery (ERAS) pathways emphasising early mobility, and in some units, prehabilitation. However, advancing age, longer duration of anaesthetic, immobility, smoking history (especially if still smoking or recently stopped) and/or an upper abdominal or thoracic incision remain key predictors of risk. Surgical patients admitted for an elective procedure will have their comorbidities optimised before admission. However, those admitted as an emergency will not—thus are at greater risk of PPCs.

AIMS

This chapter enables you to:
- Understand the surgical environment and specialities
- Assess a surgical patient
- Recognise common problems in surgical patients
- Recognise the deteriorating surgical patient and identify the early warning signs of sepsis
- Choose interventions for the surgical patient

- Understand the considerations for
  - Upper abdominal
  - Vascular
  - Orthopaedic
  - Plastic
  - Ear, nose and throat (ENT) and maxillofacial surgery, including ward-based tracheostomy
  - Patients in theatre or recovery suite

THE SURGICAL POPULATION AND ENVIRONMENT see (Table 10.1)

After extensive surgical procedures (e.g., upper abdominal surgery), patients often have multiple attachments in the early postoperative period. These include nasogastric tubes, wound drains, intravenous (IV) lines for fluids, medication or patient controlled analgesia (PCA), epidurals, central lines, total parenteral nutrition (TPN), intercostal drains, urinary catheters and supplemental oxygen. Patients from other surgical specialities have these and other attachments.

Do a 'top to toe' assessment to locate all the attachments and minimise the risk of dislodgement from moving in the bed or transferring to a chair.

TABLE 10.1 COMMON SURGICAL PROCEDURES BY SPECIALITY	
SURGICAL SPECIALTY	EXAMPLES OF PROCEDURES
Colorectal	Abdominoperoneal resection, hemicolectomy, colectomy
Upper gastrointestinal (GI)	Oesophagectomy, gastrectomy, oesophogastrectomy, pancreaticoduodenectomy
Urologic	Cystoprostatectomy, nephrectomy
Vascular	Lower limb revascularisation (e.g., femoral-popliteal bypass), aortic aneurysm repair or upper or lower limb amputation
Orthopaedic	Fracture management, joint replacement surgery
Plastics	Skin graft, flap surgery
ENT & maxillofacial	Tracheostomy, laryngectomy, facial reconstruction

Patients undergoing major upper abdominal surgery may be very weak before surgery, for example, oesophagectomy or pancreatico-duodenectomy. Nutritionally optimising these patients before surgery has a positive impact on postoperative recovery.

ASSESSING THE SURGICAL PATIENT

Find out the type, reason, date and duration of surgery, determine the extent of the incision, surgical approach and if complications arose during or after surgery. Remember patients who have returned to theatre for several operations will be more at risk of PPC.

Central Nervous System

- Major abdominal surgery is associated with high levels of pain. This impacts on diaphragm function and inhibits the patient from deep breathing, coughing and moving. Adequate analgesia is vital for assessment and performing an effective treatment
- Assess consciousness level and ability to communicate. Has this changed? Check with nursing staff if not familiar with the patient. Deteriorating levels of consciousness, engagement or confusion can be an early warning sign for sepsis ('red flag')

Cardiovascular system

- What is the heart rate/rhythm? Is it compromising blood pressure? (See Assessment Chapter 2 for normal values)
- High blood pressure may be caused by:
  - Pain/anxiety
  - Uncontrolled hypertension
- Low blood pressure may be caused by:
  - Dehydration
  - Postoperative bleeding
  - Epidural analgesia
  - Sepsis
  - Systolic blood pressure <100 mmHg is an early warning sign of sepsis

Temperature

- Pyrexia greater than 38.5° C for more than 8 hours can be caused by a lower respiratory tract infection. However, surgery itself causes reflex pyrexia with the temperature gradually rising and falling within 24 hours of operation and is not always caused by infection. Patients can be briefly hypothermic after surgery, but a temperature of less than 36º C is an early warning sign for sepsis and should be closely monitored.

Blood Chemistry

- A rise in C-reactive protein (CRP) above 10 mg/L is not always indicative of infection postsurgery. It can also be a sign of acute myocardial infarction (MI) or sepsis, which precedes pain, fever and other clinical indicators.
- A raised white blood cell count (WCC) may indicate infection (WCC $>11 \times 10^9$/L). Ethnicity directly impacts on WCC (and platelet ranges) and it may not rise in elderly patients with infection. If in doubt, seek advice from the laboratory or medical staff
- A low haemoglobin (Hb) less than140 g/L (men) or less than 115 g/L (women) may affect the ability to mobilise and may indicate blood loss

Renal System/Fluid balance
Input
- Is oral intake allowed, is the patient physically able to drink without assistance?
- Are IV fluids being given?

Output
Normal urine output (adults) = 0.5 to 1 mL/kg/h
  - Consider wound drains and insensible loss (sweat and loss of fluid from respiratory tract and gastrointestinal (GI) tract = 1 L/day. Note: insensible loss will increase by approximately 1 litre of fluid for each °C per day above 37° C)

Positive Balance (input >output)
A positive fluid balance may present in a similar way to secretion retention.
  When calculating consider:
- Blood loss in theatre
- Recent vomiting and/or diarrhoea
- Insensible loss

Causes of a positive balance may include:
- Left ventricular failure
- Cardiac arrhythmia
- Renal failure
- Profound malnutrition

Look for other signs of fluid retention before assuming a positive balance is caused by fluid overload:
- Peripheral pitting oedema (sacral oedema in the bed bound)
- Raised jugular venous pressure (JVP)
- Frothy sputum
- Dependent fine crackles on auscultation
- Chest x-ray (CXR) findings (see Chapter 4)

Be aware pulmonary oedema may coexist with a respiratory tract infection in the severely ill patient, so review the patient's sputum.

Negative Balance (output >input)
Dehydration may contribute to a sputum retention problem.

Respiratory System

Anaesthesia decreases mucociliary function, the cough reflex and reduces the ability to clear excess pulmonary secretions in proportion to the length of anaesthetic. It suppresses the sigh reflex, precipitating atelectasis. Functional residual capacity (FRC) falls because of the change of body position from upright to supine for surgical procedures, but also as a result of anaesthetic induction itself as the diaphragm and intercostal muscles relax (Saraswat, 2015).

- Respiratory rate
  - Low (<10)—if caused by morphine overdose, the patient will have pinpoint pupils. Inform ward staff immediately, this may require reversal for example, Narcan (naloxone hydrochloride)
  - High (>20)—possibly indicates pain, V/Q mismatch, acute respiratory deterioration, early warning sign for sepsis or cardiac/renal problem. Careful assessment is required. Discuss with medical/nursing teams
- Respiratory rate higher than 20 is an early warning sign for sepsis
  - Very high (>35) indicates a serious problem. Discussion with medical/nursing/outreach teams is imperative
- Respiratory pattern
  - Are there chest drains in situ? Why are they there? Are they bubbling on expiration or coughing suggesting a persistent air leak?

Is the drain connected to suction? Are they swinging (rising on inspiration and falling on expiration)? If not, is the drain blocked? (See Chapter 15 Cardiothoracic) Always check latest CXR or discuss with medical team if concerned about any changes to the drain or the patient's breathing. A repeat CXR may be required.
- Is respiratory pattern limited by pain or thoracic stiffness?
- Does thoracic expansion feel equal comparing right to left?

Arterial Blood Gases

A small deterioration in partial pressure of oxygen (PaO_2) is normal during the first 24 hours after abdominal surgery.
- Deteriorating arterial blood gases, despite increasing oxygen requirements, may signal the onset of ARDS. Very prolonged procedure (5 hours +) or major blood replacement (5 units +) are risk factors for developing this, 2 to 3 days postsurgery

Oxygen Therapy and Pulse Oximetry
- Aim to keep pulse oximetry (SpO_2) within target saturations set by the medical team. These should be documented on the drug chart. Patients with preexisting chronic lung disease may have nocturnal dips in SpO_2 for up to 5 days after surgery
- Ensure humidification in patients who have evidence of secretions and are experiencing difficulty in expectoration. It may also be useful for patients with inadequate fluid intake
  - The deteriorating patient may require more sophisticated methods of oxygen delivery to maintain SpO_2 within the appropriate range, including high flow oxygen therapy or continuous positive airways pressure (CPAP). This may require transfer to a high dependency unit or intensive care unit—consult your trust policy.

Mobilisation

Any limits to mobility? Consider:
- Drips/drains/lines
- Open abdomen, possibly with negative pressure wound therapy in situ (discuss with surgical team regarding any special instruction to ensure safety of wound during mobilisation for example, addition of a corset/support to be worn for mobilisation, or if safe to mobilise)
- CVS stability/reserve
- Respiratory stability/reserve (e.g., high oxygen requirements)

Drug Chart

If patient is nil by mouth (NBM), they may not have received their usual medication, for example a rheumatoid patient may be more immobile. Discuss with the medical team if this is the case.

Clinical Reasoning (see Table 10.2)

After surgery, the patient with a major upper abdominal incision is at risk of developing PPC if one or more of the following are present:

- Poorly controlled pain precipitating poor cough effort
- Basal or bi-basal atelectasis
- Sputum retention
- Immobility

Pain

Ensure analgesia is optimised and any assessment has included all of the aforementioned. The patient is the authority on their pain, not the clinician. If patients say they are in pain, engagement in treatment will be difficult. Check the drug chart for type/timing of medication and aim to coordinate your session with optimal pain relief. Ask the patient to move in bed, take a deep breath and cough. If they can do this, then most treatment techniques are possible. Make sure patients have had their next dose of pain relief before the effects from the previous dose have worn off. This decreases the risk of peaks and troughs in pain.

Analgesia Options

Opiates (e.g., morphine)

- Affects the central nervous system; cause drowsiness and potentially respiratory depression. Monitor respiratory rate for signs of opiate-induced reduced respiratory rate
- Oral forms of morphine (e.g., codeine) can cause constipation

Epidurals

DO NOT disconnect. Careful handling of patient is required to avoid dislodging the fine bore tube from spinal insertion, especially during transfers, standing and so on.

- Require less morphine for the same degree of analgesia, some include a local anaesthetic. Patients tend to be less drowsy or nauseous with this method but can cause itchiness
- Nursing staff may be able to adjust dosage, but if not effective over the appropriate dermatomes, a different type of analgesia is necessary

- Can result in sensory/motor loss in limbs limiting mobilisation. Check upper and lower limb sensation/movement before transfers/standing. Seek assistance from other staff if patient is weak, consider a walking aid.
- Can cause hypotension. Monitor the patient when transferring/ standing out of bed. Hypotension can cause nausea, so have a vomit bowl nearby
- May cause extreme headaches. Inform nursing/medical staff if patient complains of headache in case there is a dural tear

Patient-controlled analgesia and patient controlled epidural analgesia
- IV infusion self-administered by pressing handset, instruct to use it a minute or 2 before moving/coughing. ONLY the patient may press handset to self-administer
- It will have a 'lock out period' so they cannot receive a dose when pressing handset to prevent overdosing
- The patient chart will show how many times the device has been accessed to deliver medication and how many times they successfully received a dose. Poor delivery of patient-controlled analgesia or patient-controlled epidural analgesia will lead to poorly controlled pain and impact on physiotherapy effectiveness, discuss alternative pain relief with nursing, medical or pain team colleagues

Intramuscular Morphine
- Given as required (prn), does not give continuous pain relief—discuss alternatives with medical team if problematic.
- Intramuscular or oral analgesia takes up to 30 minutes to take effect

NonSteroidal AntiInflammatory Drugs
- Nonsteroidal antiinflammatory drugs, such as Voltarol (Diclofenac sodium) in suppository form, after colorectal surgery, may increase the risk of anastomotic leak, thus these are used with caution after general surgical procedures. In orthopaedics, dose should be effective but not be detrimental to bone healing

Paracetamol
- Paracetamol should be considered concurrently with other nonparacetamol medication as part of a multimodal approach to effective pain control. This may reduce the requirement for opiates and decrease the risk of undesirable side effects

Basal or Bi-Basal Atelectasis

FRC is reduced following abdominal surgery because of anaesthetic, pain and immobility, resulting in basal atelectasis from diaphragmatic splinting. A distended abdomen/ileus frequently leads to bi-basal compression atelectasis. If suspected, communicate with the medical team as it is vital to establish the cause.

Sputum Retention

Poor pain control, inadequate humidification during O_2 therapy, systematic dehydration and periods of being NBM, all contribute to sputum retention. Complications from specific types of surgery may lead to difficulty in expectorating because of poor cough, for example, laryngeal nerve damage following thyroid surgery.

Immobility

Immobility is a risk factor for development of PPC, deep vein thrombosis and pressure sores. Poor positioning (often slumped) in bed contributes to PPC.

Early Warning Signs of Sepsis

It is important to recognise the deteriorating patient as soon as possible. Knowing the early warning signs for sepsis is imperative.

Suspicion of deterioration or sepsis must be communicated to the nursing/medical teams, immediately as these patients deteriorate rapidly. Do not assume staff are already aware of this.

NICE (2017) Sepsis: risk stratification tools is a visual algorithm to assist clinical reasoning:

https://www.nice.org.uk/guidance/ng51/resources/algorithms-and-risk-stratification-tables-compiled-version-2551488301

Early warning signs of sepsis include:
• Temperature <36° C or >37.7° C
• Heart rate >91/min
• Systolic blood pressure <100 mmHg
• Respiratory rate >21
• New deterioration in mental status
• Decreased capillary refill time

Follow NICE NG51 (2017) Algorithm

Using the mnemonic TIME (https://www.sepsis.org/sepsis/symptoms/) may help recognition of the early warning signs of sepsis:

T—Temperature higher or lower

I—Infection – may have signs and symptoms of infection (this will also include blood results too)

M—Mental decline – confused, sleepy, difficult to rouse. A change from the previous mental state

E—Extremely ill – "I feel like I might die," severe pain or discomfort.

They also provide additional guidance for healthcare professionals regarding inflammatory, haemodynamic, organ dysfunction and tissue perfusion aspects.

Considerations in Specialist Surgical Areas (see Table 10.3)

Some surgical wards may **not be** used to dealing with patients with a compromised respiratory system.

Advise staff in the management including:

- Positioning
- Oxygen therapy
- Humidification

TABLE 10.2 INTERVENTIONS FOR COMMON PROBLEMS

PROBLEM	MANAGEMENT
Poorly controlled pain	Discuss with multidisciplinary team (MDT) to optimise analgesia When pain is controlled you can start to gain patient's trust. Explain: • the rationale behind the intervention • some discomfort is expected when deep breathing, coughing or moving • you will do as much as possible to minimise this • give the patient control • be supportive and careful when moving or handling them
Atelectasis	Good pain management and positioning in high side lying is recommended in patients with a distended abdomen/ileus. Active cycle of breathing technique is a good starting point, with positioning and hands-on for facilitation. Emphasis placed on encouraging early mobility, starting with sitting in a chair (see Chapter 6 on Management of volume loss)
Sputum retention	Causes need to be understood to optimise treatment. Good pain management and appropriate humidification, encouraging oral fluids as soon as permitted (see Chapter 5 Management of sputum). Teach the patient to support their wound for improved cough strength
Immobility	Use pillows to ensure the patient does not slip down the bed when you leave. Sit the patient out of bed and mobilise as soon as safe. In orthopaedic and plastic surgery, ascertain any specific restrictions to mobility (non or partial weight bearing) or sitting out in a chair.

TABLE 10.3 SPECIAL CONSIDERATIONS FOR SPECIALTIES	
SURGICAL SPECIALITY	SPECIAL CONSIDERATIONS
Upper gastrointestinal	Patients may have open abdomens/wounds with negative pressure dressings. Always get consultant instructions regarding mobility parameters. Do **not** use postural drainage (head down tip) after gastrectomy and oesophagogastrectomy. If cardiac (upper) sphincter of stomach has been removed, the back flow of acid may damage the anastomosis and remaining oesophagus **Always** get consultant approval before using positive pressure breathing assist devices or suctioning for patients who had a gastrectomy or oesophagostomy. These may precipitate anastomotic breakdown
Vascular	Check your trust policy for movement/mobility restrictions Arterial bypass viability: when positioning/moving patients look for: • Haemorrhage • Thrombosis • Nerve injury causing sensory/motor impairment Femoral-popliteal bypass: long incision to access arteries above and below knee. Axilla-femoral bypass: manual chest clearance techniques are **contraindicated** over the side of the graft, as the graft passes subcutaneously across chest wall Aortic aneurysm repair: breathlessness with palpable secretions may be caused by renal failure, caused by the aorta being clamped above the renal arteries during the operation, check the urine output and discuss with medical staff
Orthopaedic	Osteoporosis and fracture: A kyphotic chest may indicate collapsed thoracic vertebrae. The restricted chest movement this causes, makes this mainly elderly female group of patients highly susceptible to PPC when immobile. • Positioning is challenging, often requiring a compromise between comfort and effectiveness • Sitting out of bed/mobilising must be instituted as early as possible • Manual techniques should be undertaken with extreme caution

TABLE 10.3	SPECIAL CONSIDERATIONS FOR SPECIALTIES—cont'd
SURGICAL SPECIALITY	SPECIAL CONSIDERATIONS
	Hip Replacement: If wishing to position for optimal respiratory function. For example, forward lean sitting—discuss with surgeon. The hip may need to be flexed to >90 degrees or in high side lying the hip may be in an adducted position. Both increase the risk of dislocation External fixators: Discuss with surgeon any limitations to movement Positioning a limb with a fixator in side lying is usually possible by protecting the other limb with pillows Patients with pelvic fixators may have to remain supine, use good instruction in breathing exercises and/or adjuncts, such as mechanical insufflation:exsufflation (MI:E) or IPPB to treat effectively Rib/sternal injuries: See Chapter 15 Spinal injuries: See Chapter 14
Plastics	Dependent on site of graft there may be restrictions to movement and manual chest clearance techniques—discuss with surgeon before commencing treatment and always refer to your trust policy • No manual techniques over any type of graft affecting the chest (split skin, pedicle or free flap) • Do not change position or treat if you are unsure; ALWAYS seek advice from senior members of the team • If you spot anything you think has changed or does not look right tell the MDT—you may be the first to notice a problem!
ENT & maxillofacial	Tracheostomy: Tracheostomies may be seen in critical care or on designated tracheostomy wards. Many are temporary and patients will be able to be weaned from them before removal. A mini-tracheostomy is always temporary "On the right Trach" (2014), states all hospitals should be working towards common management goals Different trusts use different tubes—familiarise yourself with the equipment used in your facility. Trusts should also provide training for all staff involved in the management of these patients

Continued

TABLE 10.3 SPECIAL CONSIDERATIONS FOR SPECIALTIES—cont'd	
SURGICAL SPECIALITY	SPECIAL CONSIDERATIONS
	The National Tracheostomy Safety Project (NTSP) has produced bed head signs and algorithms for the management of tracheostomy (and laryngectomy) emergency. They have e-learning courses and online resources that are continually updated available at www.tracheostomy.org.uk. There is also an app for smartphones so you can have this at your fingertips! • Ensure appropriate humidification, they are at high risk of developing thick and sticky secretions as upper airway humidification systems are lost • When working with patients with a tracheostomy be aware of what tube they have, how it was inserted and the emergency algorithm to follow in the unlikely event of an emergency
	Laryngectomy: Many patients have a preoperative history of smoking, alcohol abuse and/or malnutrition, thus they are high risk for PPC • After laryngectomy, patients are solely neck breathers with no connection between the lungs and upper airways, thus their laryngectomy stoma MUST be kept clear • There may be a tracheostomy tube in place immediately postoperative BUT remember there is no connection upper airway. This tube may be sutured in place, then be replaced with a stoma button or HME and baseplate (Fig. 10.1) • Patients may retain secretions and have some postoperative bloody exudates. These are common and need to be cleared—ACBT and FET work well • It is preferable to get the patient to self-expectorate and clear with a tissue. It is possible to suction down the stoma but check your local policy • **Never** suction the tube or stoma with a yankaeur—you are blocking off the airway • Ensure appropriate oxygen delivery and humidification, they are at high risk of developing thick and sticky secretions as upper airway humidification systems are lost • Some units use an HME straight after surgery (see Fig. 10.1) • See www.tracheostomy.org.uk for management of this patient group and in particular the emergency algorithm

ACBT, Active cycle of breathing technique; *ENT*, ear, nose and throat; *FET, forced expiration technique*; *GI*, gastrointestinal; *HME*, heat moisture exchanger; *IPPB*, intermittent positive pressure breathing; *MDT*, multidisciplinary team; *PPC*, postoperative pulmonary complications.

TABLE 10.3	SPECIAL CONSIDERATIONS FOR SPECIALTIES—cont'd
SURGICAL SPECIALITY	SPECIAL CONSIDERATIONS
ENT & maxillofacial	Facial/intraoral reconstruction Takes place in specialist centres. Be aware of trust guidelines in the management of these patients. However key points to remember are: keep head in midline to avoid kinking or tension on flap • Avoid pressure from ETT tapes and trachy ties, if they are too tight, they will compromise the flap • Monitor closely, as they are high risk for postoperative complications • Do not perform respiratory techniques over the site of a new flap • Do not use yankaeur suction near an intraoral flap—you may damage the flap • Do not change position or treat if you are unsure ALWAYS seek advice from senior members of the team • How quickly complications are recognised, is directly proportional to the survival of the flap. If you spot any change or have concerns tell the MDT Communication issues: Postoperative swelling of the mouth and tongue is common and hampers communication. Try to ascertain whether the patient had communication or literacy difficulties presurgery Check they can see, hear, understand, use facial expression, such as smile/blink or write. Establish a method for the patient to indicate YES/NO—e.g., eye blink or have a picture/word/letter chart available
Theatre or Recovery suite	You may be called to recovery to a patient who has aspirated gastric contents at intubation/extubation or who has become very productive of secretions after surgery. • The theatre recovery room may have basic therapy equipment, such as airways, yankaeurs, some suction catheters and protective/sterile gloves/aprons etc • Often a lack of appropriate oxygen +/- humidification equipment available • Postural drainage is difficult/inappropriate if patient on a trolley—arrange to transfer to a bed if possible • It may be appropriate to suction the patient immediately. Theatre and recovery staff will be able to help you setting up for this

ENT, Ear, nose and throat; *ETT*, *MDT*, multidisciplinary team.

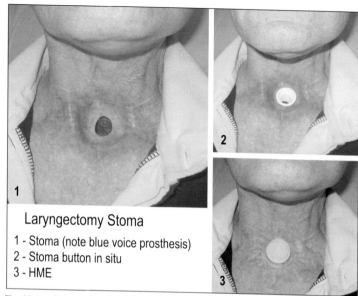

Laryngectomy Stoma
1 - Stoma (note blue voice prosthesis)
2 - Stoma button in situ
3 - HME

Fig. 10.1 • Pictures of a stoma with and without a stoma button and heat moisture exchanger from previous edition.

SUMMARY

- Comprehensive assessment enables you to identify surgical patients requiring respiratory physiotherapy, allowing for early identification of deterioration that can be feedback to the MDT appropriately
- Pain control is imperative for effective treatment of these patients
- Use www.tracheostomy.org.uk for tracheostomy/laryngectomy management

References

El-Ansary, D., Reeve, J.C., Denehy, 2016. 'Upper abdominal and cardiothoracic surgery for adults' in main and denehy. In: Cardiorespiratory Physiotherapy, fifth ed. Elsevier, Edinburgh.

Hough, 2018. 'Modifications for Different Types of Surgery' in Cardiorespiratory Care, fifth ed. Elsevier, Edinburgh.

Miscovik, A., Lumb, A.B., 2017. Postoperative pulmonary complications. Brit. J. Anaesthes. 118 (3), 317–334.

National Institute for Health and Clinical Excellence (NICE), 2017. Sepsis: Recognition, Diagnosis and Early Management (NG51) [Online] Available from: https://www.nice.org.uk/guidance/ng51/resources/sepsis-recognition-diagnosis-and-early-management-pdf-1837508256709 National Tracheostomy Safety Project [Online] Available from: http://www.tracheostomy.org.uk/.

Sepsis Alliance. Symptoms {Online} Available from: https://www.sepsis.org/sepsis/symptoms/.

Saraswat, V., 2015. Effects of anaesthesia techniques and drugs on pulmonary function. Indian J. Anaesth. 59 (9), 557–564.

Wilkinson, et al., 2014. NCEPOD On the right trach? A review of the care received by patients who underwent a tracheostomy. Available from https://www.ncepod.org.uk/2014report1/downloads/OnTheRightTrach_FullReport.pdf.

CHAPTER 11

WORKING ON MEDICAL WARDS

Jennifer Robson and Joules Lodge

INTRODUCTION TO THE MEDICAL WARDS

Medical wards deliver the majority of unplanned acute inpatient care within the National Health Services (NHS). Patients admitted for acute medical care are often complex, severely unwell or have other confounding problems. Many have multiple pathologies and require complex or protracted courses of treatment. Your role is to help manage symptoms, improve recovery time and reduce length of stay. By improving the patient's understanding and knowledge of their chronic health conditions you can help optimise symptom management, have an impact on overall health and potentially reduce the need for admission.

AIMS

By the end of the chapter you should be able to:

- Understand the medical ward environment
- Recognise common conditions and problems cared for on medical wards
- Be able to assess a medical patient
- Demonstrate clinical reasoning for the deteriorating medical patient
- Choose clinical interventions for the medical patient
- Be aware of potential contraindications and implications for physiotherapy

THE ENVIRONMENT

For optimal care, patients are admitted to speciality wards (e.g., cardiology, respiratory, renal etc) however, they may be on other wards, which can compromise communication and planning with specialist teams. On medical ward are patients with direct respiratory problems and those with indirect respiratory problems, reflecting other pathologies and comorbidities.

The Population

Some common respiratory conditions are described later, with signs and symptoms highlighted in Table 11.2 alongside the implications for physiotherapy.

Chronic Obstructive Pulmonary Disease

People with chronic obstructive pulmonary disease (COPD) may experience infective or noninfective exacerbations. An exacerbation is a sustained period of increased symptoms, not in keeping with the daily variability.

The COPD guidelines (NICE 2018) advise that all those with COPD should have a written self-management plan and should then take steps to treat their exacerbation without hospital admission. This could be through use of 'rescue packs' (oral steroids and antibiotics kept at home), or by contacting their general practitioner (GP) or primary care team. However, if they fail to improve, they then require hospital admission for more intense management.

(NonCystic Fibrosis) Bronchiectasis

People with bronchiectasis are prone to frequent infective exacerbations. They may produce lots of sputum, even when well, and should be taught airway clearance techniques, possibly including adjuncts for example, flutter to use on a regular basis at home to maintain lung health.

Cystic Fibrosis

Patients with cystic fibrosis (CF) will have a regime of mucolytics, bronchodilators and antibiotics (known as *inhaled therapies*). They will have been taught airway clearance techniques to use on a regular basis at home for maintenance of lung health and to attempt to reduce the number of infective exacerbations.

People with CF who experience frequent exacerbations should have their airway clearance techniques checked and amended as appropriate. For those who struggle to clear their airways with traditional airway clearance techniques and adjuncts (e.g., positive expiratory pressure devices), the use of noninvasive ventilation may be considered to facilitate airway clearance. It is essential that national and local trust CF infection control practices are adhered to, as patient-to-patient transmission of pathogens (e.g., *Pseudomonas aeruginosa*) has been increasingly demonstrated in this patient population.

Remember, these patients are often experts in their own management, but some do not always use their management plan! Do listen to them—they will often be able to guide you on what works best for them when they are unwell!

Interstitial Lung Disease

Patients with interstitial lung disease (ILD; patients often call this fibrosis) may experience significant shortness of breath. Initially, this is apparent on exertion, but as the disease progresses, will occur at rest. Treatment can help resolve exacerbations, but there will be a step-wise deterioration in the patient's shortness of breath and other symptoms.

Decisions regarding the ceiling of care are of importance when planning care for these patients, and early referral to palliative care teams may be appropriate to provide support and symptom management.

Asthma

It is imperative that patients with acute asthma exacerbations receive optimal medical treatment promptly. Once stabilised, their asthma management should be reviewed and adjusted appropriately. Asthma exacerbations may be triggered by a variety of factors, including allergens, pollution, smoke or exercise. Patients not responding to standard medical therapy should receive an urgent review from a senior doctor and may require discussion with the intensive care department. If you are concerned about a patient admitted with acute asthma, who is deteriorating, seek senior medical help promptly.

Pneumonia

Pneumonia is classified as either community acquired, or hospital acquired, determined according to onset of symptoms, patient factors and microbiology and these lead to different treatment strategies. The severity of pneumonia is classified according to CURB-65 (BTS 2009) with a higher score indicating greater severity and higher 30-day mortality risk (see Table 11.1).

TABLE 11.1 CURB-65		
SYMPTOM	POINTS	TOTAL SCORE
Confusion	1	Low severity 0–1 <3% mortality
Blood **U**rea nitrogen >7 mmol/L	1	Moderate severity 2 9% mortality High severity 3–5 15%–40% mortality
Respiratory rate ≥30	1	
S**B**P <90 mmHg, DBP ≤60 mmHg	1	
Age ≥**65** years	1	

DBP, Diastolic blood pressure; *SBP*, systolic blood pressure.

Patients with pneumonia, who develop respiratory failure, have a high mortality rate. Remember this, and if a patient deteriorates, seek help early! Be aware of changes in National Early Warning Score 2 and remember—a change in respiratory rate is an early marker of deterioration.

Pneumothorax
Treatment for a pneumothorax is primarily medical. It will depend on the size and impact it is having on the patient. A small pneumothorax may resolve without intervention, or simply oxygen therapy. Large pneumothoraxes require urgent management and usually an intercostal chest drain (ICD). This can be uncomfortable or painful and impacts on movement and breathing

Pleural Effusion
An accumulation of fluid between the parietal and visceral pleura. The larger the effusion, the more the respiratory system is compromised because of the inability to expand the lung. Treatment is primarily medical and often requires insertion of an ICD to drain the fluid. Common causes include malignancy, pancreatitis, liver, cardiac and renal failure

Lung Cancer
Lung cancer may be a tumour or more widespread epithelial disease. These people can be admitted to the medical ward because of an acute shortness of breath episode, which may be caused by

development of a pleural effusion or a respiratory infection for example, pneumonia. These patients may be undergoing courses of chemotherapy/radiotherapy and infection impacts on this. Decisions regarding the ceiling of care are very importance when planning care for these patients. Early referral to palliative care teams may be appropriate to provide support and symptom management (see Chapter 12 Oncology).

Hypoxaemia

Although hypoxaemia is not a pathology, the signs and symptoms and physiotherapeutic management of hypoxaemia is included in Table 11.2, as it is a common problem occurring across many pathologies and warrants specific physiotherapy consideration.

NONRESPIRATORY PATHOLOGIES THAT CAN IMPACT ON RESPIRATORY FUNCTION

Some common nonrespiratory conditions are described subsequently. Table 11.3 highlights the signs and symptoms, and implications for physiotherapy.

Heart failure

Heart failure can occur as a consequence of severe cardiac or respiratory disease and is commonly managed with diuretics. Associated dependent oedema can affect peripheral sensation and balance mechanisms, impairing mobility.

Acute Myocardial Infarction

Patients admitted following an acute myocardial infarction may only be on the ward a few days, whilst waiting for transfer to another unit, and will only need intervention if they have other associated respiratory or mobility problems. Be guided by your local trust protocols.

Pulmonary Embolus

This is a blood clot in the pulmonary arterial circulation preventing perfusion of part of the lung. Treatment for pulmonary embolus is usually therapeutic anticoagulation, but in some cases, the patient may undergo a procedure to remove the clot.

TABLE 11.2 COMMON PROBLEMS IN THE MEDICAL RESPIRATORY PATIENT

PROBLEM	COMMON SIGNS AND SYMPTOMS FOUND ON ASSESSMENT	PHYSIOTHERAPY TREATMENT CONSIDERATIONS
Noninfective exacerbation of chronic lung disease	• ↑WOB • Breathlessness • Dry cough • Fatigue • Hypoxaemia • Hypercapnia	• Breathlessness management and pacing (see Chapter 7) • Airway clearance techniques (see Chapter 9) • Maintenance of mobility • Referral to pulmonary rehabilitation • Referral to community COPD/respiratory teams
Infective exacerbation of chronic lung disease including COPD, bronchiectasis and CF	• ↑WOB • Breathlessness • Productive cough • Hypoxaemia • Hypercapnia • Fatigue • Chest pain • Temperatures • Hypoxaemia • Hypercapnia	• Airway clearance techniques, • Medication review—e.g., check inhaler technique, mucolytics • Noninvasive ventilation may be indicated in acidotic type 2 respiratory failure (see Chapter 8) • Time treatments appropriately with any nebulised medication • Referral to pulmonary rehabilitation
Interstitial lung disease (ILD)	• Breathlessness • Fatigue • Hypoxaemia • Respiratory infection	• Oxygen • Breathlessness management strategies, pacing and education • Noninvasive and invasive ventilation is not appropriate in those with severe disease
Asthma	• Bronchospasm • Respiratory infection • ↑WOB • Anxiety **If severe,** • Hypoxaemia • Hypercapnia	• Medical management with nebulised bronchodilators • Airway clearance techniques • Positions to ease breathlessness • Correction of breathing pattern • Breathing control/diaphragmatic breathing • Nose breathing • Relaxation techniques, e.g., visualisation

Continued

TABLE 11.2	COMMON PROBLEMS IN THE MEDICAL RESPIRATORY PATIENT—cont'd	
PROBLEM	COMMON SIGNS AND SYMPTOMS FOUND ON ASSESSMENT	PHYSIOTHERAPY TREATMENT CONSIDERATIONS
Pneumonia	• ↑WOB • Breathlessness • Productive cough • Inspiratory crackles • Bronchial breathing • Fatigue • Chest pain • Temperatures • Hypoxaemia • Hypercapnia	• Oxygen & humidification therapy • Positioning for optimal V/Q matching • Mucolytics • Airway clearance techniques • PEP adjuncts • Breathlessness management and pacing • Mobilisation
Pneumothorax	• Absent breath sounds on affected side • Tracheal deviation • ↑WOB • Unequal chest expansion • Chest pain of sudden onset • Hyperresonant percussion note	• Thoracic expansion exercises • **Do not** lift a chest drain higher than the site of insertion!Ensure careful handling of ICD on exercise and movement • Mobilisation—always gain approval to remove patients ICD from wall suction if necessary • Pain may affect lung expansion and patient's function. Consider analgesia and patient education on posture and upper limb movements • Pneumothorax should be excluded or treated before any positive pressure treatment
Pleural effusion	• ↓Breath Sounds • Dull percussion note • ↑WOB • Breathlessness • Chest pain • Unequal chest expansion	• Breathlessness management and pacing • Small pleural effusions may not require drainage • For patients with a chest drain, see advice under pneumothorax • Encourage mobilisation • Thoracic expansion exercises

TABLE 11.2	COMMON PROBLEMS IN THE MEDICAL RESPIRATORY PATIENT—cont'd	
PROBLEM	**COMMON SIGNS AND SYMPTOMS FOUND ON ASSESSMENT**	**PHYSIOTHERAPY TREATMENT CONSIDERATIONS**
Lung cancer	• Cough – dry/productive • Haemoptysis • Breathlessness • ↑WOB • Fatigue • Pain • Clubbing	• Breathlessness management and pacing • Positions of comfort or to ease breathlessness • Airway clearance techniques • Cough control • Mobilisation • Oxygen • (see Oncology Chapter 12)
Hypoxaemia	• ↑WOB • Breathlessness • Tachycardia • Peripheral and/or central cyanosis	• Causes of transient hypoxaemia may include sputum plugging, partial/total airway obstruction, or hypoventilation • Oxygen has a drying effect on the mucous membranes and therefore those requiring high flow rates should be considered for humidification • Supplemental oxygen should be prescribed to target saturations (see Respiratory failure Chapter 8) • In an emergency, oxygen should be given without a prescription, but this should be addressed when the patient stabilises

CF, Cystic fibrosis; *COPD*, chronic obstructive pulmonary disease; *ICD*, intercostal chest drain; *PEP*, positive expiratory pressure; *WOB*, work of breathing.

Pulmonary Oedema

If the left ventricle 'fails' as a pump, blood backs up in the veins of the pulmonary circulation. The increase in pressure in the blood vessels pushes fluid into the alveoli, which disrupts normal oxygen transfer across pulmonary membranes. Pulmonary oedema can be from cardiac or noncardiac origins.

TABLE 11.3	COMMON PROBLEMS IN THE MEDICAL NONRESPIRATORY PATIENT	
PROBLEM	COMMON SIGNS AND SYMPTOMS FOUND ON ASSESSMENT	PHYSIOTHERAPY TREATMENT CONSIDERATIONS
Heart failure	↑WOB Breathlessness Nonproductive cough Dependent oedema Hypoxaemia	• Breathlessness management and pacing • Mobility assessment and provision of walking aids • Oxygen therapy
Pulmonary embolus	↑WOB Breathlessness Haemoptysis Chest pain Hypoxaemia	• Breathlessness management and pacing • Mobility is only considered once therapeutic anticoagulation is achieved • Pain may limit normal thoracic expansion Consider appropriate analgesia
Pulmonary oedema	↑WOB Breathlessness, particularly when lying flat Cough, productive of frothy white/pink stained sputum	• Breathlessness management and pacing • Airway clearance techniques are not appropriate in pulmonary oedema
Haemoptysis	Cough, productive of fresh blood ↑WOB Hypoxaemia	• Airway clearance techniques may continue to be beneficial in those with an infection and associated small amounts of haemoptysis • Moderate to large volume haemoptysis is a contraindication to the use of positive pressure. It is advisable to use an alternative airway clearance technique in these patients • Consideration should be made to positioning of patients. Consider high side lying with the bleeding side down • Prompt review of those with large/massive volume haemoptysis is critical

TABLE 11.3	COMMON PROBLEMS IN THE MEDICAL NONRESPIRATORY PATIENT—cont'd	
PROBLEM	**COMMON SIGNS AND SYMPTOMS FOUND ON ASSESSMENT**	**PHYSIOTHERAPY TREATMENT CONSIDERATIONS**
Renal failure	↑WOB Breathlessness	• Breathlessness management strategies may be of limited use as the increased respiratory rate is caused by the metabolic acidosis, requiring respiratory compensation
Pancreatitis	↑WOB Breathlessness Abdominal pain and distention Reduced basal air entry	• Breathlessness management and pacing • Lung expansion may be affected by pleural effusions and ascites. Encouraging deep breathing and mobility to avoid further complications • Pain may limit thoracic expansion. Consider appropriate analgesia
Oesophageal varices	Cough/vomiting fresh blood	• Airway clearance techniques in those with concurrent lung infection or chronic sputum production • Avoid excessive coughing
Osteoporosis	Pain Skeletal deformities loss of height Bone fractures	• Caution should be taken with 'hands on' therapy because of the increased risk of fractures • Encourage weight bearing exercise to improve musculoskeletal strength, consider falls reduction programmes
Immuno compromise	Recurrent infections	• Airway clearance techniques in those with an infection or with chronic mucous production • You need to understand local infection control policies. Those with severe immunocompromise may require reverse barrier nursing to reduce the risk from contracting illnesses/infections from other patients

WOB, Work of breathing.

Haemoptysis

Bleeding from the airways occurs because of:
- Infection (e.g., tuberculosis, pneumonia)
- Pulmonary embolus
- Clotting disorders/anticoagulation use
- Lung cancer
- Cardiac disorders
- Trauma, for example, pulmonary contusions

Small amounts or streaky haemoptysis can worry patients but are unlikely to need specific treatment. Moderate or larger amounts of haemoptysis may need specific treatment.

It is important to ask patients about frank haemoptysis and document it.

Renal Failure

Renal failure may be acute (also known as *acute kidney injury* or *AKI*), chronic or acute-on-chronic. Chronic kidney injury is not reversible.

The kidneys and lungs have a role in maintaining the acid-base balance in the blood. If either system is compromised, the other must compensate to avoid acidosis or alkalosis. In AKI, there is potential for metabolic acidosis, which will be compensated by respiratory drive being increased, producing hyperventilation and a fall in partial pressure of carbon dioxide (pCO_2) to restore pH to normal. Therefore people with AKI can present with an increased respiratory rate, despite normal oxygenation, and an absence of other respiratory signs.

Pancreatitis

Inflammation of the pancreas, either acute or chronic, results in nausea, vomiting and upper abdominal pain. Do not assume all patients are alcoholics because pancreatitis can also be caused by gallstones! Acute pancreatitis can be very severe, and patients may require critical care, but the symptoms can be reversed, chronic pancreatitis is not reversible.

Oesophageal Varices

These are dilated veins in the lower third of the oesophagus that develop as a consequence to portal hypertension most commonly from cirrhosis of the liver. These enlarged veins can bleed (severely), especially with increased pressure, for example, from coughing. Blood from this type of bleed or coming from the stomach is called *haematemesis*.

Osteoporosis
Loss of bone density is natural with aging but can be severe in some people, especially those who smoke or drink heavily, or those who need recurrent or long-term steroids.

Immunocompromise
Immunocompromise can be the result of immunological disorders (chronic conditions, such as diabetes, hepatitis, or human immuno-deficiency virus [HIV], some cancers) and also through the use of immunosuppressants (chemotherapy, medications for ILD and rheumatoid arthritis and posttransplant immunosuppression). Inhibition of the body's natural defences' mechanisms leads to an increased risk of infection and potentially slower recovery.

It is important these patients are educated on the importance of maintaining good general health and fitness. Immunocompromised patients may be offered antiviral or antibiotic treatment at a lower threshold than those who are immunocompetent.

PHYSIOTHERAPY ASSESSMENT OF THE MEDICAL PATIENT

Central Nervous System
Chest pain, from cardiac, thoracic or musculoskeletal causes, impacts on the function of the diaphragm or inhibits the patient moving and/or coughing. Adequate analgesia is essential for effective assessment and treatment. Although excessive opioid analgesia may supress respiratory drive and affect consciousness, low dose opioids can be useful in managing symptoms of breathlessness.

Cardiovascular System
Some commonly used drugs, such as salbutamol and theophylline, can cause tachycardia and cardiac rhythm disturbances. Continuous

heart rate/rhythm monitoring is advised during intravenous theophylline use.

Renal/Fluid Balance

A positive fluid balance may lead to pulmonary oedema and/or peripheral oedema.

A negative fluid balance can cause airway secretions to become thicker and more difficult to expectorate.

Patients on oral mucolytics (e.g., carbocisteine) should be encouraged to stay well hydrated (unless there is medical advice to restrict fluid intake) to maximise their effectiveness.

Respiratory System

Respiratory Pattern

Patients with severe emphysema may not be able to demonstrate diaphragmatic breathing because hyperinflation produces a flattened diaphragm. Their breathing pattern is likely to comprise apical expansion with accessory muscle use.

Chest expansion may be unilaterally affected in those with a pleural effusion or pneumothorax. Severe lobar pneumonia can also cause poor expansion of the affected lobe, leading to asymmetry in chest wall movement.

Auscultation

Remember, those with chronic lung disease are not likely to have normal breath sounds on auscultation, even when they are well. Patients with severe emphysema can have extremely quiet and sometimes inaudible breath sounds and patients with other conditions may have widespread crackles and polyphonic wheezes every day.

Sputum

Those with chronic lung disease may always have sputum. You should enquire about change in quality (colour, consistency) and quantity, as this may guide assessment and treatment.

Reduced sputum volume, in those with ongoing symptoms of infection, is often a sign of difficulty clearing or plugging rather than improvement.

It is worth considering whether a sputum sample should be sent for culture and sensitivity to identify the cause of infection and guide antibiotic treatment.

Arterial Blood Gases

People with chronic lung or heart disease are likely to have 'abnormal' arterial blood gases as their 'normal' because of chronic hypoxaemia and/or hypercapnia. In general, a partial pressure of oxygen (PaO_2) of 7.3 kPa or higher is tolerated in those with chronic lung conditions like COPD. However, if there is a secondary problem, such as polycythaemia, cor pulmonale or pulmonary hypertension, then PaO_2 should be 8kPa or more.

SPECIFICS OF PHYSIOTHERAPY TREATMENT OF THE MEDICAL PATIENT

Oxygen Therapy and Pulse Oximetry

(See Chapter 8 Respiratory failure and BTS Guidelines [BTS, 2017])

The deteriorating patient may require more sophisticated methods of oxygen delivery to maintain pulse oximetry (SpO_2) within the target range, including high flow oxygen therapy, continuous positive airways pressure (CPAP) or bilevel positive airways pressure (BiPAP). This may require transfer to high dependency or intensive care unit.

Patients may require supplemental oxygen when mobilising, even if they do not at rest. Monitor SpO_2 during and for a period of time after a mobility assessment to ensure there are no associated desaturations. A drop in SpO_2 of more than 4% from the patient's baseline to below 90% indicates the need for ambulatory oxygen, which needs prescription.

Exercise and Pulmonary Rehabilitation

Exercise and activity increase tidal volume and can decrease peripheral oedema by improving venous return using the muscle pump.

Postexacerbation pulmonary rehabilitation (within 1 month of discharge from hospital) is beneficial to those with chronic lung disease, it reduces the risk of readmission, improves quality of life and exercise capacity (NICE 2018).

Airway Clearance

People with chronic respiratory conditions may have already been taught airway clearance techniques previously. Check their usual practice and make appropriate changes to technique and/or frequency.

They should be encouraged to continue their usual airway clearance methods, unless there is a contraindication. It may be appropriate to add positive expiratory pressure devices, inspiratory positive airway pressure devices, manual physiotherapy techniques, or a combination of these (Treatments see Chapter 9).

Medication

Inhaler technique should be reviewed regularly, as there is a high incidence of errors in use, even in patients who have used devices since childhood. There are also extremely high rates of inhaler errors in healthcare professionals, so it is imperative a competent person assesses technique. There are two main types of inhaler device, metered dose inhalers (MDIs) and dry powder inhalers (DPIs), which require different inspiratory techniques. A spacer can improve drug deposition to the lungs with MDI devices, and their use should be encouraged. DPIs generally require a higher inspiratory flow rate than MDIs (although this varies between specific devices) so they may not be effective in acute exacerbations or as disease progresses.

Mucolytics—carbocysteine or hypertonic saline (NaCl 7%) are frequently used in these patients to help thin secretions and aid expectoration. Commencing them or optimising the dose during admission could be beneficial.

Some medications, such as antiparkinsonian medications, should be given on a strict schedule to ensure their effects are optimised. If patients are on these medications, consider their impact on their ability to participate in therapy.

End-of-Life Care/Ceiling of Care

Chronic medical conditions are life limiting. Frequent admissions to hospital may indicate a progression of disease or increasing frailty and nearing the end of life. Best practice is to ensure that resuscitation status is discussed with all patients and the outcome clearly documented. It is good practice for these discussions to also consider ceilings of care, that is the extent of treatment that is deemed appropriate and, in the patient's, best interests.

Palliative care includes symptom management and is not just about end of life management. Patients can be referred for palliative care support at any stage in their disease, depending upon their response to treatment and their symptom burden.

Anxiety Management

Chronic health conditions are strongly associated with anxiety and depression. Patients with chronic lung conditions associate their breathlessness with their underlying condition rather than their mental health. This can lead to increasing use of medications, which may not improve symptoms. Depression leads to social withdrawal and associated reduction in activity and exercise, leading to reduced cardiovascular fitness and further breathlessness, in a vicious cycle of inactivity.

Referral to support and psychological services may be beneficial to the patient. Disease specific support groups (e.g., Breathe Easy—see reference list) or charities may be able to offer patient education and emotional support to promote self-care and improve quality of life.

Stress Incontinence

This can be a common problem for people with chronic cough. Muscle weakness in the pelvic floor, combined with increased pressure from coughing, can lead to urinary incontinence. This is a significant problem for the patient, but they be too embarrassed to seek help. Teaching pelvic floor exercises is a good starting point – using sustained holds and short contractions, also 'the knack'—that is, contracting the pelvic floor before coughing. Leaflets on these exercises may be available in your Trust or a referral to a women's health physiotherapist can be considered if more specialist advice is needed. 'Squeezy' is an NHS physiotherapy app for pelvic floor muscle exercises that may be helpful.

Breathlessness and Anxiety

Breathlessness and anxiety are a significant problem for these patients, frequent experience of unpleasant symptoms give rise to distress (see Work of Breathing—Chapter 7).

Key Messages

Physiotherapy has a significant, varied role in treating the medical patient.

Thorough assessment will clearly identify the patient's problems and appropriate treatment strategies.

Knowledge of other major systems builds understanding of their impact on the respiratory system.

References

National Institute for Health and Care Excellence, (NICE). 2018 Chronic Obstructive Pulmonary Disease in over 16s: diagnosis and management NICE. Guideline. www.nice.org.uk/guidance/ng115.

British Thoracic Society (BTS), 2009. Guidelines for the management of community acquired pneumonia in adults update 2009, Available from: https://www.brit-thoracic.org.uk/document-library/clinical-information/pneumonia/adult-pneumonia/a-quick-reference-guide-bts-guidelines-for-the-management-of-community-acquired-pneumonia-in-adults/.

British Thoracic Society (BTS), 2017. Guideline for oxygen use in healthcare and emergency settings, www.brit-thoracic.org.uk/standards-of-care/guidelines/bts-guideline-for-emergency-oxygen-use-in-adult-patients/.

Breathe easy information available from https://www.blf.org.uk/support-for-you/breathe-easy.

Further Reading

National Institute for Health and Care Excellence (NICE) (2018) Chronic heart failure in adults: diagnosis and management, www.nice.org.uk/guidance/ng106.

National Institute for Health and Care Excellence (NICE) (2017) Asthma: diagnosis, monitoring and chronic asthma management, www.nice.org.uk/guidance/ng80.

National Institute for Health and Care Excellence (NICE) (2017) Cystic fibrosis: diagnosis and management, www.nice.org.uk/guidance/ng78.

https://www.cuh.nhs.uk/breathlessness-intervention-service-bis.

CHAPTER 12

WORKING ON ONCOLOGY

Katherine Malhotra and Jess Whibley

INTRODUCTION

Cancer is treated in three ways: surgery, radiotherapy and chemotherapy. Often, these are used in combination to provide the most effective treatment.

Cancer treatment depends on the site of the primary cancer, histology and the stage of disease when diagnosed. You need to be aware that many older patients with cancer may have poor health, before treatment, because of comorbidities, which increases the risk of respiratory complications and impact on their ability to comply with physiotherapy interventions.

Newly diagnosed patients may lack an understanding of their current disease and it is essential to be aware what they and their relatives/next of kin know about the diagnosis. Many have high anxiety levels and may fear dying, this must be considered before seeing the patient.

AIMS

By the end of the chapter you should have:

• Greater awareness of issues pertinent to a person with cancer
• Better understanding of terminology to assist you assess and review medical records

THE ENVIRONMENT

Oncology patients are in all healthcare settings; including surgical and medical wards, critical care, outpatients and emergency care.

Some are treated in isolation, in a single-occupancy room to reduce the spread of pathogens and help additional infection control precautions, such as reverse barrier nursing, which protects the patient from the environment. It is essential you adhere to your trusts infection control policy.

THE POPULATION

Patients with a cancer diagnosis and respiratory complications need assessment and intervention. Their respiratory symptoms may be as a result of the cancer itself, or its treatment (e.g., surgery, chemotherapy). Often the respiratory presentation will be very similar to patients and conditions you have encountered before. For example, a patient with a diagnosis of gynaecological cancer may be in hospital with an exacerbation of chronic obstructive pulmonary disease.

Specifics of Assessment

Be confident you understand Chapter 2 Assessment before continuing.

General
- Is this a sudden/gradual change in condition?
- Where is the cancer, primary site, evidence of secondary spread?
- Stage of treatment, that is, acute/palliative
- Resuscitation status of patient/ceiling of treatment identified and clear in the notes
- Are they limited by pain, fatigue, nutritional status?
- Are they in isolation (haematology or neutropenic patients) and reverse barrier nursed to protect them from infection?

Central Nervous System
- Any signs of altered level of consciousness, possibility of brain metastases?
- Is the respiratory drive affected?
- What sedatives/medications are they taking/receiving?

Cardiovascular
- Cardiovascular stability, including arrhythmias and support, including inotropes and vasopressors?
- Are they exhibiting signs of sepsis (Surgery—see Chapter 10)
- Consider the risk of rapid deterioration, especially in haematology patients
- What are the blood results? Are they on anticoagulation medication? Are they actively bleeding? It is quite common for oncology patients, particularly those with a haematooncological malignancy, to have low platelets which puts them at risk of bleeding (See Appendix 2 -normal values tables)

Respiratory
- Are there signs of chest disease not related to cancer?
- Could there be a tumour obstructing the airways?
- Could there be fibrotic or interstitial changes?
- Could this be an atypical infection (particularly in haematology patients)?
- Is there a pleural effusion?

Musculoskeletal
- Do they have bony metastases? Will this affect you mobilising the patient or undertaking respiratory techniques? Ensure you are not causing pain to the patient and that they have adequate pain relief before using manual techniques or mobilising. Check any mobility restrictions with the multidisciplinary team.
- Is there a possibility of spinal cord compression? Refer to local trust policies in line with the National Institute of Health and Care Excellence (NICE) guidance regarding manual handling of these patients (NICE 2014).

Clinical Reasoning

These patients present with similar problems to other respiratory patients, including breathlessness, increased work of breathing and sputum retention (see Chapters 5–7). The clinical reasoning issues, in the management of oncology and haematology patients, relates to the treatments that they are having, the complications of the disease and the stage of treatment; anywhere from active care to end of life management. (Treatments—see Chapter 9).

Clinical Interventions

For patients presenting with respiratory problems secondary to:
- Bone marrow depression
- Acute oncology
- Metastatic oncology
- End of life care

Potential interventions and considerations for treatment are highlighted, as well as identifying when physiotherapy may not be appropriate in Tables 12.1 to 12.4.

TABLE 12.1 BONE MARROW DEPRESSION

- Side effect of chemotherapy
- Increased risk of infection
- More common with blood cancers (leukaemia, myeloma and lymphoma)
- Includes neutropenia (low white cell count), thrombocytopenia (low platelet count) and anaemia (low haemoglobin)

Common issues	Advice
Neutropenia and Neutropenic sepsis	Neutropenia: • A low white cell count (<0.5 × 10^9 L) • Makes it difficult to mount a normal response to infection. The patient may present with an unproductive cough and ↑ work of breathing, use positioning to assist breathing control Neutropenic sepsis: • Temperature above 38° C • A low white cell count (<0.5 × 10^9 L)
Thrombocytopenia **Hazard**	• A low platelet count (<150 × 10^9 L) • Platelets prevent bleeding and a low count is the commonest cause of bleeding in haematooncological patients • Patients who are febrile or septic do not maintain platelet levels and require extra support with platelet transfusions • All hospitals should have a policy for when to transfuse • In general, platelets are transfused when levels have dropped between 10–20 × 10^9/L • Physiotherapy interventions should take place during or immediately after platelet transfusion • Liaise with medical team regarding target platelet count and patient's normal range These patients can be treated but require extreme caution. If you are unsure ask for help! • Need to know platelet count • Need to know if actively bleeding • Minimise intervention if actively bleeding, i.e., positioning and breathing exercises • If requiring suction, ensure count above 20 × 10^9/L (check local policy/seek medical advice) • Can suction whilst platelets being transfused • Manual techniques, i.e., percussion and vibrations can be used to assist with sputum clearance, if no other option to aid clearance Use a towel to decrease risk of bruising and ensure patient comfort

TABLE 12.1   BONE MARROW DEPRESSION—cont'd

Anaemia	• A low haemoglobin (Hb) count (<135 g/L in men and <115 g/L in women) • Anaemia occurs in haematooncological malignancies because of decreased red cell production, the primary disease process or blood loss from surgery • Most centres attempt to keep a patient's Hb level >80 g/L • Patients may present with shortness of breath on exertion because blood is unable to carry sufficient oxygen to the body's muscles, therefore increasing demand on the respiratory system and increasing the work of breathing (see Chapter 7). • Physiotherapy is not appropriate, medical management should reverse symptoms

TABLE 12.2   ACUTE ONCOLOGY

COMMON ISSUES	ADVICE
Tumour occluding airway	• Primary lung cancer may cause airway obstruction, atelectasis +/- consolidation behind the tumour and inflammation around the tumour • Patient may have stridor, requiring urgent medical intervention • Patient may sound productive • Physiotherapy is not appropriate to clear secretions from behind a tumour • Ensure good positioning to reduce the work of breathing, O2 therapy, adequate analgesia and monitor • Physiotherapy may be appropriate after primary therapy has shrunk the tumour

Continued

TABLE 12.2	ACUTE ONCOLOGY—cont'd
COMMON ISSUES	**ADVICE**
Mucositis	• Inflammation of mucosa of mouth and throat is a common side effect during and after chemotherapy ± radiotherapy • Excessive production of thick, mucoid upper respiratory tract secretions with mouth soreness and ulceration are common • Patients find it difficult to clear secretions and can be at risk of aspiration • Mucositis can be mistaken for chest infection • Advice on breathing exercises and use of high volume forced expiration techniques to clear upper airway • Avoid Yankaeur suction if possible as it may exacerbate symptoms • Regular mucolytic/hypertonic saline nebulisers may help break down secretions, making them easier to clear (refer to your local trust policy) • Chest infection may coexist and should be treated accordingly
Aspergillosis	• Opportunistic fungal infection • Occurs with prolonged neutropenia or severe bone marrow depression • Bronchopulmonary aspergilloma can cause cavitating lesions and invade arterioles and small vessels • Symptoms include malaise, weight loss, fever and productive cough ± haemoptysis • If infective sputum present use airway clearance techniques, including gentle manual techniques • No physiotherapy if frank haemoptysis is present
Pneumocystis carinii pneumonia (PCP)	• Opportunistic infection in immunocompromised patients causing inflammation in the lungs • Organisms damage the alveolar lining and produce a foamy exudate • Symptoms include a dry cough, increased respiratory rate, breathlessness, hypoxemia and fever • Auscultation may reveal fine, diffuse crackles • X-ray usually shows a haze in the hilar region developing into diffuse symmetrical shadowing (butterfly) • Medical treatment is O2 therapy, respiratory support and antibiotics • Physiotherapy advice on positioning for relaxation, breathing control and mobilisation may help

TABLE 12.2 ACUTE ONCOLOGY—cont'd	
COMMON ISSUES	ADVICE
Pneumonitis	• Inflammatory condition which may be progressive • Radiation-induced, drug related or of viral origin, e.g., cytomegalovirus, respiratory syncytial virus (RSV) • Patients have a dry cough, increased respiratory rate and breathlessness • Medical treatment is with high dose steroids in acute stages • In self-ventilating patients, RSV is treated with nebulised ribavirin (Vitrazole) This nebuliser presents a HAZARD—wear appropriate personal protection equipment, including facemask (see your local trust policy for administration instructions) • Physiotherapy advice on positioning for relaxation and breathing control may help
Disseminated intravascular coagulation	• A bleeding disorder with an alteration of the blood clotting mechanism • Caused by an underlying disease process (always a secondary condition) • Major causes in this population are severe sepsis and acute promyelocytic leukaemia • Caution with physiotherapy interventions because of risk of haemorrhage, no manual techniques

TABLE 12.3 METASTATIC ONCOLOGY	
COMMON ISSUES	ADVICE
Spinal cord compression hazard	• Caused by primary or metastatic cancer by extradural or intradural compression on spinal cord • An oncology emergency - treatment (if appropriate) surgery, radiotherapy or occasionally chemotherapy is vital to minimise neurological deterioration • Can occur at any spinal level, characterised by motor and sensory loss below level of compression with bladder and bowel changes • Patients may experience respiratory difficulties depending on level of compression. Abdominal muscles can also be compromised reducing the patient's ability to cough

Continued

TABLE 12.3	METASTATIC ONCOLOGY—cont'd
COMMON ISSUES	**ADVICE**
	• Physiotherapy options depend on stability of the spine, condition of patient and pain control • Be aware of trust protocols, especially if repositioning • Check with doctors regarding stability of spine before physiotherapy (see Chapter 14) • Interventions can include positioning, active cycle of breathing technique, assisted cough and intermittent positive pressure breathing, if indicated (see Chapter 9)
Bony metastatic disease hazard	• Often associated with pain, can lead to pathologic fracture and hypercalcaemia • Common in breast cancer, prostate cancer, lung cancer and myeloma patients • Usually affects long or flat bones of skeleton • Check for the presence of bony disease before chest physiotherapy using x-rays/scan reports if available • Adequate analgesia should be administered before treatment • Gentle one-handed percussion can be used if necessary, with a towel for cushioning • Use chest vibrations (even if rib metastases are present) if no other technique is successful for sputum clearance • Rib fracture may occur—CAUTION • Ensure patient can express their discomfort/pain
Hypercalcaemia	• Increased serum calcium levels usually associated with presence of bony metastatic disease • Symptoms include confusion, lethargy, nausea and vomiting, constipation and thirst • You need to be aware of this condition as symptoms can compromise effective treatment
Pleural effusion	• Excessive amount of fluid in pleural space • Symptoms include pallor, cyanosis, dyspnoea, increased respiratory rate, decreased breath sounds and dullness on the affected side, decreased pulse oximetry (SpO2) and chest pain • Pleural effusion can be identified on chest x-ray

TABLE 12.3	METASTATIC ONCOLOGY—cont'd
COMMON ISSUES	**ADVICE**
	• Causes collapse of the surrounding lung tissue • Medical treatment includes thoracocentesis/pleural tap or insertion of intrapleural drain (see Chapter 11 Medical)
Superior vena cava obstruction	• Primary or metastatic cause • Caused by external compression or internal obstruction of the superior vena cava • Associated with lung cancer with direct compression from a mass in the right main bronchus or lymphoma, with compression from the mediastinal or paratracheal lymph nodes • Presents with swelling of neck, upper trunk, upper extremity, dyspnoea with hypoxia, cough and chest pain • Medical treatment is essential with radiotherapy or chemotherapy • Physiotherapy not appropriate
Ascites	• Excessive fluid in peritoneal cavity • Symptoms abdominal distension and discomfort, nausea and vomiting, leg oedema, and dyspnoea • Medical treatment is with drugs and drainage of peritoneal cavity via a catheter (paracentesis) • Ascites will compromise diaphragmatic excursion • Positioning will be difficult • Physiotherapy is not appropriate • Advice on forward lean sitting/side lying may help
Lymphangitis carcinomatosa	• Diffuse infiltration of lymphatics of lungs by cancer cells • Symptoms include dyspnoea, cough ± pleuritic chest pain and central cyanosis • Medical treatment is with drug therapy (corticosteroids and O2 therapy) • Physiotherapy not appropriate • Advice on positioning may help to assist breathing control

TABLE 12.4   END OF LIFE CARE

Ceilings of care may depend on tumour and symptom burden. As a result, a patient may not be for resuscitation or interventions, such as invasive ventilation or escalation to critical care. They may still benefit from your input to manage their respiratory compromise.

Be aware that ceilings of treatment may not be indicative of end of life.

Common issues	Advice
Death rattle	• A rattling noise produced by secretions in back of throat oscillating in time with inspiration and expiration • Can be distressing for relatives, carers and other patients • Antisecretory agents are useful, e.g., glycopyrronium or hyoscine • Physiotherapy is not appropriate but explanation that patient is not distressed may ease families' anxieties • Advice regarding positioning may be beneficial • Do not encourage suction as it can increase secretions further
Terminal restlessness	Common in period immediately preceding death Use of sedation may be necessary to keep patient comfortable

Physiotherapy intervention is limited in these stages, but you could refer to, or liaise with, palliative care or symptom control team for review.

It can be distressing you may feel helpless in these situations, but you must recognise your professional limitations

Seek support from peers

EQUIPMENT

Some specific pieces of equipment are often used in the cancer setting. These include:

Hickman Catheter
• Used for long-term venous access
• Tunnelled under the skin, a catheter is introduced via the subclavian vein and exits midway from the anterior chest wall
• The tip lies in the superior vena cava or right atrium

Peripherally inserted central catheter line
• Inserted into one of the large veins of the arm near the elbow

- A long, thin, flexible catheter is slid into the vein until the tip sits in a large vein just above the heart
- The peripherally inserted central catheter line can be used to give chemotherapy, antibiotics, intravenous fluids and nutritional support.

Syringe Driver
- Portable battery-operated infusion pump
- Used for a continuous administration of drugs via a subcutaneous route
- Used for analgesics, antiemetics, dexamethasone and anxiolytic sedatives

Epidural Infusion (Via an In-Dwelling Spinal Catheter or IntraThecal Catheter)
- Epidural analgesia is administration of analgesics into epidural space
- Used for postoperative pain control or treatment of chronic intractable pain

Note
Check blood counts
Patients fatigue quickly so keep treatments short
Consider analgesia and do not forget the importance of positioning for patients in pain
Modify treatments if bony metastatic disease and be aware of risk of spinal cord compression
Position for breathlessness and increased work of breathing; do not rush!
End of life care: think about comfort

Recommended Reading
Dougherty, L., Lister, S., 2015. The Royal Marsden Hospital Manual of Clinical Nursing Procedures, ninth ed. Blackwell Science Ltd, Oxford.

Grundy, M., 2006. Nursing in Haematological Oncology, second ed. Bailliere Tindall, London.

Hoffbrand, A.V., Shaw, P.A.H., 2015. Essential Haematology, seventh ed. Wiley Blackwell, Oxford.

Macmillan, 2018. Physical Activity Guidelines for People with Metastatic Bone Disease. Macmillan, London. Available at: https://www.macmillan.org.uk/_images/physical-activity-for-people-with-metastatic-bone-disease-guidance_tcm9-326004.pdf.

NICE, 2014. Metastatic Spinal Cord Compression In Adults. Available at: https://www.nice.org.uk/guidance/qs56.

Walshe, C., Preston, N., Johnston, B., 2017. Palliative Care Nursing: Principles and Evidence for Practice, third ed. Open University Press, London.

CHAPTER 13

WORKING ON THE CRITICAL CARE UNIT

Susan Calvert and Amy Bendall

INTRODUCTION

The critical care unit (CCU) can be daunting initially, but it is one of the safest places to work with knowledgeable staff and information readily available on charts and monitors to support you to make good clinical decisions.

You may find critically unwell patients located elsewhere in the hospital and some hospitals have critical care outreach teams to support this. This chapter will only describe the physiotherapeutic care provided on CCU.

AIMS

By the end of this chapter you will be able to:

- Identify key differences in assessing a patient on CCU compared with a patient on a ward
- Interpret common attachments/monitoring in CCU and their significance for physiotherapy
- Identify specific considerations in physiotherapy care on CCU

THE CRITICAL CARE ENVIRONMENT

In critical care, there may be many types of equipment, medications, alarms and noises that are unfamiliar. If so, use the expertise of the bedside nurse who can help you. Alarms sound frequently in critical care – look to see what the cause is and determine if any immediate action is required. Liaise with the bedside nurse and always check before silencing alarms.

Even if a patient is sedated, continue to talk to them as if they are awake. Every effort should be made to facilitate communication with patients. In patients who are even slightly awake, use communication

TABLE 13.1	CLASSIFICATION OF CRITICAL CARE
Level 0	Patients whose needs can be met through normal ward care in an acute hospital
Level 1	Patients at risk of their condition deteriorating, or those recently relocated from higher levels of care, whose needs can be met on an acute ward with additional advice and support from the CCU team
Level 2	Patients requiring more detailed observation or intervention, including support for a single failing organ system, postoperative care and those 'stepping down' from higher levels of care *Requires a minimum of 1:2 nursing staff ratio*
Level 3	Patients requiring advanced respiratory support alone, or basic respiratory support together with support of at least two organ systems. This includes all complex patients requiring support for multiorgan failure *Requires a minimum of 1:1 nursing staff ratio*

Guidelines for the provision of Intensive Care Services; Edition 1.1 2016

strategies, such as asking closed questions, pen and paper, pointing charts and alphabet boards to help.

Classification of critical care indicates the dependency that individual patients have, regardless of location in the hospital (Table 13.1.)

Core standards for CCUs in the United Kingdom recommend a closed unit model of intensive care, where care is led by a consultant in Intensive Care Medicine, as this has been shown to improve mortality and morbidity. Some hospitals separate people needing 'high dependency' (level 2) from those needing 'intensive care' (level 3), others look after both levels in the same unit.

The Population

The patients in CCU depends on hospital size and specialist services provided. Essentially, any admission to hospital can deteriorate and require more advanced interventions. Table 13.2 summarises commonly seen clinical presentations on CCU (see Chapters 14 and 15 for cardiothoracic and neurologic specifics).

Sepsis

Sepsis is a common cause of admission to CCU. This is a syndrome of physiological, pathological and biochemical abnormalities induced by

TABLE 13.2	COMMONLY SEEN CLINICAL PRESENTATIONS ON A CRITICAL CARE UNIT	
	SPECIALITIES	COMMON CONDITIONS
Medicine	Respiratory, cardiology, endocrinology & diabetes, gastroenterology, hepatology	Community acquired pneumonia, out of hospital cardiac arrest (OOHCA), diabetic keto-acidosis, decompensated alcoholic liver disease
Surgical and cancer	Elective or emergency, upper and lower gastrointestinal (GI), urology & renal, vascular, oncology & haematology	Oesophagogastrectomy, laparotomy (e.g., hemicolectomy), cystoprostatectomy, nephrectomy, amputation, neutropenic sepsis
Trauma and orthopaedics	Elective or trauma	Total hip/knee replacement, spinal surgery, fractured ribs, polytrauma, for example, after road traffic incidents

infection. Any of the conditions in Table 13.2 can be complicated by sepsis.

Go back to "Early warning signs of sepsis" (see Chapter 10 Surgery) and familiarise yourself with National Institute for Health and Care Excellence (NICE) NG51 (2017) algorithm and trust guidelines for sepsis in your trust.

SPECIFICS OF PHYSIOTHERAPY ASSESSMENT

Clinicians take different approaches to assessment—The A to E approach works well in acute situations, ensuring a logical order is adopted. Chapter 2 Assessment offered you this and a different systems-based assessment approach; see which you feel works best for you or follow the system recommended in your trust.

A—Airway

Patients will either be self–ventilating (SV) or have a 'supported airway', such as an endotracheal tube (ETT) or tracheostomy. For those with a supported airway check:

- *Is the airway patent?* Can you pass the suction catheter fully? Do they have an end tidal CO_2 (EtCO2) trace (see later)? With a tracheostomy, check the inner tube
- *Is the airway in the correct position?* Numbers on the side of the ETT show depth of insertion. Check it has not been pushed in or pulled out as this could affect the patient's ventilation

B—Breathing

If the patient is on a ventilator, do not over complicate this! Look – listen – feel – think.

What you would assess in a spontaneously breathing patient: are oxygenation and ventilation adequate? (See Chapter 2 Assessment).

When listening to a ventilated patient's chest, consider the extraneous noises, for example, water in the ventilator tubes, air leak around the cuff. Sometimes when a patient is being delivered breaths at tidal volumes, and/or has a high positive end expiratory pressure (PEEP), there is reduced turbulence in the airflow, so added sounds are less obvious, making the chest sound clear. To assess for retained secretions, expiratory vibrations and chest wall palpation can be helpful in this situation.

Differences in Monitoring on Critical Care

- *Pulse oximetry*: If a patient is peripherally shut down (without a good peripheral blood supply) pulse oximetry (SpO_2) monitoring will be via an ear probe or headband instead of a finger probe. Probes should only be used for the areas they are designed for. Otherwise readings may be inaccurate.
- *Capnography*: The $EtCO_2$ can confirm the correct position of the airway and provide a trend suggesting if ventilation is improving or worsening (arterial blood gases [ABGs] should confirm this).

Mechanical Ventilators

There are lots of different ventilators, familiarise yourself with the equipment your unit uses during your induction. Common concepts apply to most ventilated patients:

- *Control versus support.* In control mode, the patient makes no effort; the ventilator controls all elements of breathing. In a support mode, the ventilator assists the patient's own efforts.
- *Pressure versus volume.* If pressure is controlled, then volume will vary depending on lung compliance (i.e., how easily the lungs fill). Alternatively, if volume is controlled then pressure will vary according to compliance.
- *PEEP.* A Splinting pressure that helps hold the lungs open during expiration to improve oxygenation. Avoid disconnecting the patient from the ventilator if PEEP is more than 10 cmH2O.
- *Pressure support or peak airway pressure* shows how much help (pressure) a patient is requiring on inspiration. If lung compliance falls, more pressure is needed to ensure adequate ventilation.

C—Circulation (see Chapter 2 Assessment for more details)

- *Heart rate*: three electrocardiogram (ECG) leads (red, yellow, green) give a basic ECG trace. Look for normal sinus rhythm, is it regular? Check with the nurse or doctor if you see unusual patterns or rates.
- *Blood pressure* (BP). is often monitored invasively by an 'arterial line' placed in the radial or femoral arteries. Consider very high or very low readings, as well as those unusual for the patient. *Mean arterial pressure* is considered a better indicator of organ perfusion than systolic BP and this is often recorded and referred to on CCU.
- *Temperature*: this may be artificially controlled, for example, following out of hospital cardiac arrest OOHCA to lower the metabolic rate or when a dangerously high temperature is present. Ice packs or an intravascular heat exchange catheter, which circulates cold water through a line inserted into the femoral vein, may be used.
  If hypothermia is present (especially if undergoing renal replacement therapy), a warming blanket may be used.
- *Supportive medication*: Vasoactive drugs for example, dobutamine (Inotrope); noradrenaline, vasopressin, metaraminol (vasopressors) can be used to support BP if it is low. Note the amount/dose and if these infusions are increasing, static or decreasing—this indicates cardiovascular stability and can guide you regarding precautions or contraindications to interventions.
- *Fluid balance:* Calculation of difference between fluid input and fluid output will be recorded on charts and provides information about hypovolaemia (when fluid output exceeds input) and hypervolaemia (when fluid input exceeds output). Urine output is a guide to renal perfusion and cardiac output. This is regularly measured in CCU—see normal values for target ranges (Appendix 2).
- *Central venous pressure*: is measured via a central venous catheter inserted via the internal jugular or subclavian vein. This reflects the amount of blood returning to the heart and the pressure in the right atrium. For example, it would be decreased with hypovolaemia.
- *Other invasive monitoring* (e.g., pulse index contour continuous cardiac output, inter aortic balloon pump, pacing wires [See *cardiothoracic chapter 15*]).

D—Disability

If the patient is critically unwell, assessment of neurological status is commonly the focus, with assessment of musculoskeletal function completed as the patient clinically improves. However, do not forget the impact that restricted range of movement and altered muscle tone will impact on physiotherapeutic interventions to improve cardiorespiratory function (e.g., positioning to improve ventilation/perfusion (V/Q) and/or drainage of retained secretions). Therefore consideration of musculoskeletal function is necessary – even in the very unwell patient.

An assessment of a patient's neurological status (see Chapter 2 Assessment) should be completed as necessary for the patient's clinical presentation.

Considerations in Critical Care

- *Consciousness level* can be assessed using the Glasgow Coma Scale (GCS); when intubated the maximum verbal response is 1 (because the patient will be unable to produce a sound). This automatically reduces intubated patients' GCS to 11, even if they are completely alert. The quicker tool 'AVPU' score is often used (see Chapter 2 Assessment).
- *Cooperation level* can be assessed by Standardised Five Questions (SQ5). This involves asking the patient to undertake five different tasks (e.g., open and close your eyes). Each correct answer is worth 1 point (a patient fully awake and cooperative will achieve a score of 5). This is a useful measure of when you would assess voluntary muscle strength and evaluate mobilisation options.
- *Use of sedation* aims to minimise patient distress and maximise the efficiency of MV to facilitate extubation as soon as possible. Common sedatives are benzodiazepines (e.g., Midazolam) and propofol, which are often combined with analgesics (e.g., morphine and fentanyl) to reduce pain, improve ETT tolerance and reduce dyspnoea.
- On CCU, the Richmond Agitation and Sedation Score (RASS) is commonly used. The sedation scoring system used in your unit will be on the charts for you to refer to and interpret.
- *Delirium* is characterised as a disturbance of consciousness and cognition that develops over a short period and fluctuates over times. The Confusion Assessment Method for the intensive care unit (CAM ICU) is commonly used to identify this. Take delirium into account when planning your interventions.

- *Neuromuscular blockade (paralysing)* agents (e.g., atracurium) facilitate intubation, minor procedures, invasive ventilation, and can lower intracranial and intraabdominal pressure. Negative side effects include: increased risk of critical illness polyneuropathy; reduced cough reflex and post traumatic stress disorder.
- *Invasive monitoring*, such as intracranial pressure (ICP) bolts are used to measure the pressure in the brain after a serious neurologic injury (see Chapter 14 Neurological).
- *Spinal stability.* Spinal injury may cause a neurological deficit. Strict handling and positioning guidelines exist to protect the spinal cord from further damage. If in doubt treat as an 'unstable' injury (see Chapter 14 Neurological).

E—Exposure

Consider other body systems or information not already covered. Because exposure of the patient's body is often required to gather information, ensure their dignity and comfort is maintained at all times.

- *Laboratory investigations*: Commonly seen haematological and biochemical results include: haemoglobin (Hb); white blood count (WBC); platelets (PLTs); activated partial thromboplastin (APTT); international normalised ratio (INR); sodium; potassium; urea; creatinine: c-reactive protein (CRP); lactate; bilirubin; albumin. Familiarise yourself with the significance of these results for physiotherapy—this list is not exhaustive and there may be others pertinent to specific conditions that you need to understand.
- *Abdomen*: Some conditions cause abdominal distension; this restricts basal expansion and can lead to volume loss. Look for hernias, stomas, percutaneous endoscopic gastrostomy (PEG) feeding tubes, as you need to modify handling/moving accordingly.
- *Body habitus*: Consider body mass index—respiratory function is affected by obesity and malnourishment for different reasons. Both extremes need to be considered with manual techniques or total body positioning. See also 'ideal body weight' for ventilation
- *Nutrition*: Nasogastric (NG) tubes are commonplace in CCU because of disturbances in gastrointestinal function and/or inability for oral intake. PEGs and nasojejunostomy tubes are used to facilitate enteral feeding (through the gut) or total parenteral nutrition (directly into the blood via the central line) can be used.
- *Other considerations:* Check wounds and drains for evidence of fluid loss or bleeding; ask the nurse about other fluid loss (e.g., diarrhoea) or bleeding.

CLINICAL REASONING: PUTTING IT ALL TOGETHER

Consider each assessment finding and what it suggests (see Chapters 5–8). Remember, be logical and consider what problems physiotherapy can help, when precautions/contraindications may preclude physiotherapy interventions, or if the problem requires medical/surgical management only.

Clinical Interventions

Many interventions used with patients on the ward are applicable to CCU. The simplest interventions, for example correct positioning, are often the most effective (see Chapter 9 Treatments).

Sometimes, physiotherapy treatment is not required, for example, if a patient has an effective cough and secretions are clearing easily on suction, additional input would not be required, unless the secretions compromise the patient's respiratory function or clear less effectively. Ensure advice is given about positioning, use of adjuncts (e.g., humidification) and that the patient is monitored for changes in their condition that may necessitate reassessment and treatment.

In CCU, where patients can be unstable, try to change one thing at a time. For example, if you reposition the patient into left side lying, do not start a nebuliser simultaneously as it could be unclear what has made a difference. Make a change whilst monitoring the patient closely, and once you are happy that they are stable, continue with additional interventions.

Treatments for Sputum Retention

- *Positioning for $\dot{V}/\dot{Q}$ matching and postural drainage.* Ventilator care bundles advise positioning a patient with the head up 30 degrees. Avoid head down tilting. Consider pausing enteral feed and emptying NG tubes to avoid aspiration. Remember, when a patient is on a ventilator (or any positive pressure device), air will follow the path of least resistance, therefore, in side lying, the nondependent (top) lung will have better ventilation.
- *Suction* can be performed relatively easily in a ventilated patient if an 'in-line suction catheter' or 'closed suction system' is present, as this minimises disconnection time from the ventilator. Open suction is also commonly used on critical care units. Ensure you familiarise yourself with your trust policy regarding these procedures.

- *Manual techniques* can cause incorrect ECG readings. Stop the technique and check the ECG reading returns to its normal rhythm before recommencing.
- *Cough augmentation* maybe required to manage sputum retention (see Chapter 9).
- Nebulisers can be administered to a ventilated patient using a T-piece connector.
- Humidification of the ventilator circuit can be passively enhanced using a heat moisture exchange unit. This is a filter that collects the heat and moisture on the patients' exhalation, this is then picked up and returned to the patient on the next inspiration delivered. Active humidification can also be achieved using a heated water vapour system at the optimal temperature of 37° C at the mouth.

Treatments for Reduced Lung Volumes

- *Positioning:* Upright positions promote increased lung volumes. If a patient is stable enough, mobilisation out of bed is the simplest way to improve lung volume. Multiple attachments and tubes should not be a barrier to mobilisation, however, careful risk assessment and planning is required to ensure mobilisation is achieved safely. In the very hypoxic patient, prone positioning may be used to help the posterior/dorsal areas of the lung reexpand and optimise $\dot{V}/\dot{Q}$ matching.
- *Active cycle of breathing technique* and *intermittent positive pressure breathing* can be used in the treatment of reduced lung volumes (with SV and awake patients). Manual hyperinflation (MHI) or ventilator hyperinflation produces similar effects in a ventilated patient. If you are not competent and confident in these procedures, discuss with a senior doctor or nurse, who will be able to perform the technique for you, while you undertake positioning, manual techniques and suction.
- *Removal of the cause* of reduced lung volumes: for example sputum clearance or reducing external compression of the chest (e.g., abdominal distention secondary to constipation or ascites).

Treatment Considerations

- *PEEP greater than 10*: Avoid disconnection of the ventilator circuit (e.g., for MI-E or MHI) and long/repeated suctions because this causes loss of the pressure splinting the lungs open, producing increasing alveolar collapse and worsening oxygenation.

- *Acute respiratory distress syndrome* is an acute inflammatory lung injury. It affects the lungs in a heterogeneous pattern; thus some alveoli will be stiff, uncompliant and thickened, making gas exchange more difficult, whilst other alveoli are unaffected. To avoid injuring unaffected alveoli and worsening affected alveoli, low tidal volumes and a high PEEP are used with MV. In these patients, hyperinflation techniques should be avoided as the positive pressure moves predominantly to the unaffected alveoli, which are more compliant and causes over distention.
- Ensure there are no precautions/contraindications to physiotherapy interventions. For example, coagulopathy (e.g., low platelets); flail chest; loss of skin integrity (e.g., burns/skin grafts); increased or labile intracranial pressure; cardiovascular instability. These need to be taken into account, and treatments modified or not completed, depending on the clinical presentation. Senior physiotherapy staff and members of the multidisciplinary team (e.g., CCU consultant/nurse) can support junior physiotherapists by discussing the clinical presentation and supporting clinical decision making.
- Mobilisation improves respiratory function, psychological wellbeing and promotes functional independence. It should therefore be used where clinically able. There are a number of published algorithms and guidelines providing guidance and consensus on when it is safe to complete mobilisation. Included within these are: the physiological assessment of the patient, the consideration of attachments (e.g., invasive lines and monitoring), the management of sedation and environmental factors. During your induction, familiarise yourself with NICE CG83 (2009) guidelines and Quality Standard [QS158] for the rehabilitation of adults after critical illness and any specific protocols or guidance in your trust regarding early mobilisation of patients on CCU.

Evaluating Outcomes

Identify markers which gauge whether physiotherapy interventions have been effective. Examples of objective markers commonly used in CCU include: SpO2; fraction of inspired oxygen (FiO_2); ABGs, ventilator settings and auscultation findings. If the patient is responsive and able to communicate, then patient-centered parameters are also useful, for example assessment of pain (e.g., visual analogue scale) and breathlessness (e.g., modified BORG dyspnoea scale).

In addition, there are a number of different functional measures for use with critically ill patients that have undergone clinimetric evaluation, for example Physical Function in Intensive care Test scored (PFIT-s); Chelsea Critical Care Physical Assessment tool (CPAx); ICU Mobility Scale (IMS). These are useful to provide baseline information and measure functional change.

Treatment on CCU often needs to be short and focused, do not be afraid to finish a treatment session when you have identified improvement(s) in objective marker(s). If there is no identifiable change in the patient's presentation after treatment, go back to your assessment and ensure you have not missed anything. Review the problem list to see if there are other treatment technique(s) that may be more effective.

After treatment, think carefully about when you will review the patient next. Ask yourself: *when would the physiotherapy service usually review this patient and, based on your clinical reasoning, do you need to come back sooner?* Physiotherapy on CCU is often timed around: personal care; changing the patient's position for pressure care; nebulisers and any other procedures that may be taking place.

There are other occasions where a patient does not respond to physiotherapy interventions as expected. The bedside nurse will support you and you might ask the doctors to review. Stop physiotherapy at that point and await their opinion.

Make sure you record your interventions using the correct documentation for the unit you are working in. Verbally feedback to the bedside nurses, what you found, what you did and when you are planning to review again.

References

Levels of Critical Care for Adult Patients, 2009. Intensive Care Society. Available at: https://www.ics.ac.uk.

Core Standards for Intensive Care Units ed 1, 2013. Faculty of intensive care medicine. Available at: https://www.ficm.ac.uk.

National Institute for Health and Clinical Excellence (NICE), 2009. Rehabilitation after critical illness in adults clinical guideline [CG83]. Available from: https://www.nice.org.uk/guidance/cg83.

National Institute for Health and Clinical Excellence (NICE), 2016. Sepsis: Recognition, diagnosis and early management (NG51). [Online] Available from: https://www.nice.org.uk/guidance/ng51/resources/sepsis-recognition-diagnosis-and-early-management-pdf-1837508256709.

National Institute for Health and Clinical Excellence (NICE), 2017. Sepsis: risk
    stratification tools. Available from: https://www.nice.org.uk/guidance/ng51/resour
    ces/algorithm-for-managing-suspected-sepsis-in-adults-and-young-people-aged-18-
    years-and-over-in-an-acute-hospital-setting-2551485715.
National Institute for Health and Clinical Excellence (NICE), 2017. Rehabilitation after
    critical illness in adults quality standard [QS158]. Available from: https://www.nice.
    org.uk/guidance/qs158.

CHAPTER 14

WORKING ON THE NEUROSURGICAL/ NEUROLOGY UNIT

Kate Jones

INTRODUCTION

Injury or disease affecting the nervous system affects the respiratory system in several ways:

- Problems affecting the respiratory centre impact on rate, pattern and depth of ventilation.
- Insults to the brain, the spinal cord or the nerves innervating the respiratory muscles affect the ability to swallow, breathe and cough.
- These result in reduced lung volumes, retention of secretions, increased work of breathing and respiratory failure.

These patients often appear stable, because of compensation, for a period of time (especially if young) but deteriorate rapidly if warning signs are not observed. They must be monitored carefully, and appropriate action taken quickly if required. Good monitoring produces, good management—seek help from colleagues if you are unsure or have concerns.

AIMS

By the end of the chapter you will be able to:

- Assess and decide whether to treat, or not, a patient with neurological impairment
- Know who to ask for information
- Know when to request additional help

THE POPULATION

Acute Brain Injury

An acutely brain injured patient is usually cared for in specialist environments (neurosurgical/trauma critical care). Patients are comprehensively monitored by an expert team, so any deterioration in respiratory parameters can be detected promptly.

Spinal Cord Injury

A patient with new high cervical injury (above C5) is likely to require ventilation assistance and cared for in level 2 or 3 environments, high dependency or critical care. Patients with injuries in the thoracic or lumbar regions, are less likely to require ventilatory assistance, but this also depends on age and other comorbidities. New spinal cord injury (SCI) patients are ideally managed in a specialist spinal unit whereas longstanding/established SCI patients are more likely to be found on a general ward in a local hospital where staff may not be as familiar with management of this patient group.

Neuromuscular Disorders

Neuromuscular weakness can be acquired (e.g., Guillian Barré Syndrome [GBS] and Motor Neurone Disease [MND]) or congenital (e.g., the dystrophies). These patients are at risk of respiratory problems because of any combination of immobility, reduced airway protection, progressive inspiratory and expiratory respiratory muscle weakness. If admitted to hospital, there may be no clear diagnosis, and they may be admitted to nonspecialist wards. If monitoring is inadequate, deterioration may be undetected, and the risk of respiratory failure significant.

Assessment in NeuroLogical Injury

Respiratory decline in neurological patients is linked to:

- Decreased inspiratory muscle function secondary to changes in muscle innervation (more likely in SCI or neuromuscular disorder).
- Altered respiratory drive from disturbances in central functioning (more likely in the neurosurgical patient because of postoperative/injury swelling or a direct injury to the brain).
- Reduced airway protection, or poor swallow—often referred to as *altered bulbar function.*
- Physiological responses to a neurological injury, including altered mechanics of breathing, hypersecretion, bronchospasm and pulmonary oedema. These compound the other problems.

Acute traumatic neurological patients (e.g., SCI or head injury) frequently have other injuries that impact on respiratory function and limit treatment options for example, chest, abdominal or facial injuries.

These changes in respiratory mechanics can lead to sputum retention, volume loss, increased work of breathing, and ultimately respiratory failure. Your assessment needs to be thorough and detailed to ensure these patients' respiratory functions are optimised (see Chapter 2 Assessment and Chapter 8 Respiratory failure). Nursing staff caring for these patients, over one or more shifts, will know the 'normal' trends in observations for them and what has prompted the need for a respiratory intervention.

Specific assessment in this population are trends or changes in:

- Intercranial pressure (ICP)—that is, pressure within the cranium
- Cerebral perfusion pressure (CPP) —that is, blood flow to the brain
- Mean arterial pressure (MAP)
- Glasgow coma scale (GCS)
- Pupils; size, shape, reactivity to light and equality
- Forced vital capacity (FVC) and peak cough flow (PCF)
- Spinal shock and autonomic dysreflexia in spinal injuries
- Anxiety
- Pain
- Drains, wounds, for example, extra ventricular drains, craniectomy (see Clinical reasoning section)
- Respiratory observations
  Some parameters are only be measured in specialist units

Intracranial Pressure

Direct Intracranial Pressure Monitoring
Prolonged elevations in ICP are secondary to one or more of:

- Hypoxaemia and/or hypercapnia (both increase vasodilation within the brain)
- Increased cerebral oxygen consumption for example, fitting, hyperglycaemia, increased temperature
- Increased cerebral inflammation/oedema
- Expanding intracerebral, subdural or extradural haematomas
- Hydrocephalus that is, where cerebrospinal fluid flow is obstructed
  A prolonged increase in ICP can result in compression of the brain stem, potentially forcing it through the foramen magnum. If not corrected quickly, this damages the respiratory centres, cranial nerves and ultimately leads to brain stem death. Normal values for ICP are less than 15 mmHg, a critical value is 25 mmHg or higher (i.e., capillary pressure).

Without ICP monitoring, other signs of increased ICP are:
- Severe headaches
- Altered vision, change in pupil size/reactivity
- Vomiting
- Hypertension
- Bradypnoea, abnormal respiratory pattern of alternating rapid shallow breaths, apnoea and deep breathing
- Bradycardia
- Systolic hypertension, bradycardia and bradypnoea are termed *Cushing's triad* – a late sign that there may be significant pressure on the medullary centres of the brainstem

Cerebral Perfusion Pressure

CPP relates to the blood flow to the brain, it determines brain perfusion. Normal values for CPP are 60 to 70 mmHg.

$$CPP = MAP - ICP$$

$$e.g.\ MAP(70) - ICP(10) = CPP(60)$$

An ICP above 25 mmHg means inadequate blood flow to the brain, a low CPP and secondary damage to the brain because of cerebral ischaemia.

A good blood pressure is also important as if MAP is low, CPP will also be lowered.

Physiotherapy is to maximise gaseous exchange without compromising CPP.

Target Values in Acute Head Injury Patients

PARAMETER	RANGE
Temperature	36° –37.5° C
Mean arterial pressure	>90 mmHg
Partial oxygen pressure	>11 KP$_a$
Partial pressure carbon dioxide	4.0–5.0 KPa
Blood glucose	6–10 mmol/L
Sodium	140–155 mEq/L
Cerebral perfusion pressure	60–70 mmHg
Serum osmolarity	290–310 mosmol/L

Brain Trauma Foundation Guidelines, 2016. accessed at https://braintrauma.org/uploads/07/04/Guidelines_for_the_Management_of_Severe_Traumatic.97250__2_.pdf

Glasgow Coma Scale

A drop in GCS indicates potential physiological deterioration. A persistent and/or unusual drop in GCS requires urgent medical review and potentially emergency intervention. A GCS of less than 8 is a significant concern because of the risk of airway compromise and requires senior medical review.

Information on GCS can be found at https://www.glasgowcomascale.org/

Pupils

Changes in reactivity, size or equality of the pupils directly reflects changes intracranially. This could be caused by raised ICP and medical advice should be sought.

Forced Vital Capacity and Peak Cough Flow

These measurements are important objective markers in patients with neuromuscular disease who have respiratory muscle weakness, indicating lung volumes and cough effectiveness. Measure with a spirometer and a peak flow meter, ideally in a consistent position. Serial measurements are vital, providing trends. If measurements show FVC is falling, this can indicate fatigue or deterioration in neuromuscular strength. Values that are falling rapidly or are below 1.5 L warrant urgent medical review. An FVC of less than 1 litre may mean a patient needs transfer to critical care, if this is not above their ceiling of care.

Cough strength correlates well with the noise generated. If PCF falls below 270 L/sec, and an infection is suspected or confirmed, cough augmentation should be considered. When PCF falls below 160 L/sec, cough augmentation is essential.

Special Considerations for the Spinal Injured Patient

Immediately following a traumatic SCI, there is period of spinal shock resulting in a flaccid paralysis below the level of injury. For the intercostal muscles, this creates an unstable chest wall. During inspiration, the negative intrathoracic pressure causes the paradoxical inward depression of the ribs, that is, your ribs move inward during inhalation rather than outward. This mechanical imbalance causes less efficient ventilation and respiratory compromise.

Within the first 24 to 48 hours postinjury spinal shock, which is swelling, can progress up the spinal column, producing paralysis above the level of the injury. This is significant in a patient with a cervical injury, as the respiratory muscles, most notably the diaphragm, can be further compromised. Monitoring of FVC and PCF are of paramount importance at this time. Patients can fatigue and develop type 2 respiratory failure very quickly (see Chapter 8 Respiratory failure).

Autonomic Dysreflexia
In acute SCI injuries at T6 or above, there is a high risk of autonomic function being compromised, resulting in significantly altered blood pressure and heart rate. In established SCI, this altered autonomic function can lead to a **potentially life-threatening condition** called *autonomic dysreflexia*. This is caused by any noxious stimulus below the level of the spinal injury. Bladder or bowel distention, pressure areas and infection are all common causes. Symptoms include hypertension, bradycardia, pounding headache, flushing, sweating or blotching above the level of injury but pale and cold below.

Fatigue
Respiratory muscle fatigue in spinal patients can be overlooked; they can deteriorate rapidly necessitating urgent intervention.

Anxiety
Minimising anxiety and fear is important to optimise respiratory function. This can be difficult to manage, particularly in acute illness. Building trust and rapport with the patient is essential as the psychological impacts of these injuries should never be underestimated.

Pain
Pain can be a important. There may be an obvious source of pain or generalised discomfort because of immobility. This will affect their ability to ventilate, comply with treatment and increase their fear and anxiety.

Respiratory Observations
Important observations in the spinal/neuromuscular patient are:
* Respiratory rate and volume
* Respiratory pattern – spinal patients may have paradoxical breathing

- Cough efficiency
- Voice quality—do they have a "wet" voice? Are they able to speak clearly?

Clinical Reasoning

Common respiratory problems, singly or in combination, include:
- Sputum retention
- Lobar collapse/volume loss
- Increased work of breathing
- Respiratory failure

NEUROSURGERY PATIENTS

What is the patient's response to suction or coughing and handling/procedures?
- Does **ICP** rise? By how much?
- **Does CPP** fall? By how much?
- How long does the ICP/CPP take to settle?

ICP normally rises on coughing but returns to a resting level within seconds. When considering treatment, the time taken for the ICP to settle is a key factor identifying if your patient is low, medium or high risk (Table 14.1).

If your patient does not have ICP monitoring and their vital signs are affected by suction, coughing, handling or other procedures AND takes longer than 5 minutes to return to normal – classify them as high risk.

The phrase 'maximum involvement; minimal intervention' is used with these patients. So, if your patient is in the high-risk group, you must be confident that you can improve gaseous exchange by

TABLE 14.1	ASSESSING PATIENT'S RISK		
RISK	ICP	CPP	PATIENT STABILITY ON INTERVENTION
Low	< 15	70	All parameters stable
Medium	15–20	70	ICP rises with intervention but settles quickly within few minutes
High	>20	<70	If your patient is sensitive on interventions, ICP rises and takes >5 minutes to settle

CPP, Cerebral perfusion pressure; *ICP*, intercranial pressure.

TABLE 14.2 POINTS OF CONSIDERATION IN THE MANAGEMENT OF NEUROSURGICAL PATIENTS

POINT OF CONSIDERATION	SOLUTION/CONTRAINDICATION
Extraventricular drains or lumbar drains	Do not change bed height Drains may need to be clamped before treatment Check local policy
Recent craniectomies	Patients with no bone flap should not be rolled onto that side
Unsecured aneurysms/newly secured aneurysms	Check with medical team what level of mobility/cough is acceptable before treating
Transphenoidal patients	Check with the medical team if allowed to cough
Fractured base of skull	No suction without a protected airway
Fear/anxiety/cognitive difficulties	Discuss patient's response to new situations/people/interventions with the multidisciplinary team

removing secretions and/or re-inflating a collapsed area. Optimise the situation and proceed with care, always discuss with colleagues if you are unsure.

Neurosurgical patients may have other postoperative precautions of note (Table 14.2).

PATIENTS WITH A CERVICAL SPINAL INJURY

Consider the stability of the injury, if in doubt **always** treat as unstable. Use a head hold for all interventions and log rolling for repositioning. Follow trust policies and consult the multidisciplinary team (MDT). Be mindful of additional injuries in polytrauma patients.

What Is the Level of Injury?

Table 14.3 summarises the effect of SCI on muscle groups and vital capacity. Higher injury equal more respiratory compromise, including

	EFFECT ON	
TABLE 14.3	**RESPIRATORY FUNCTION IS DEPENDENT ON LEVEL OF INJURY**	

LEVEL	EFFECT ON RESPIRATORY MUSCLES	VITAL CAPACITY IN ACUTE STAGE (% OF NORMAL)
C1–C2	Partial innervation of accessory muscles	5%–10% (500–600 mL)
C3–6	Accessory muscles and some/all diaphragm	20%–30% (1 litre)
C7–T4	Accessories, diaphragm and partial intercostals	30%–50% (1380–2300 mL)
T5–T10	Diaphragm, accessories, partial intercostals, partial abdominals	75%–100% (4–5 L)

Chin, L.S., 2018. Spinal cord injuries. Accessed at: https://emedicine.medscape.com/artic le/793582-clinical

cough. Patients may require cough augmentation techniques (see Chapter 9 Treatments).

Hypotension and episodes of bradycardia may affect how you manage this patient

Positioning

Patients with high SCI ventilate better in supine. FVC rises because of the abdominal contents pushing the diaphragm up. Do not try to sit these patients to help them breathe more easily, the opposite is the case! Note the degree of abdominal distension, when the patient last had their bowels open as they are at risk of paralytic ileus—which will contraindicate manual assisted cough.

How Long Ago Was Their Injury? see (table 14.4)

Patients with established SCI tend to deteriorate rapidly when fatigued. They are very aware of what works for them, so listen to the patient/carers when planning treatment.

TABLE 14.4 CONSIDERATIONS IN SPINAL CORD INJURY

POINT OF CONSIDERATION	SOLUTION/CONTRAINDICATION
Established diagnosis	Patients/carers will be aware what treatments are most beneficial Is there regular physiotherapy and a care plan identifying when to use cough augmentation and noninvasive ventilation
New/unknown diagnosis	Fear and anxiety may be an issue Chart respiratory function closely to identify deterioration
Ceiling of treatment	Be aware of advanced management plans and your role
Pattern of deterioration	Signs of bulbar weakness appearing Reducing motor power
Positioning restrictions	Does tone/body deformities limit positioning
Fear/anxiety/cognitive difficulties	Multidisciplinary team consideration of how patient copes with new situations/people/interventions

Respiratory rate is an early marker of change. Watch out for the patient who has a climbing rate that then seems to settle, this is often a sign they are fatigued and reaching their limits of compensation (see Respiratory failure Chapter 8).

NEUROMUSCULAR PATIENT

Considerations in the management of neuromuscular patients (Table 14.4)

TREATMENTS

There are some special treatment considerations with this group (see Management Chapters 5–8 and Treatment Chapter 9) see Table 14.5

TABLE 14.5	PATIENT PROBLEMS AND PHYSIOTHERAPY INTERVENTIONS	
PROBLEM	**CONSIDER**	**PHYSIOTHERAPY INTERVENTIONS**
Sputum retention	• Can the patient protect their airway? • Is cough effective?	• Positioning and appropriate humidification are vital • Manual techniques (must be bilateral and in supine for acute cervical spinal cord injury) • Breath stacking, manual assisted cough or manual in/exsufflation (MI:E) can all be used prophylactically
Volume loss	• Good supported positioning is vital • Is there appropriate seating/positioning equipment? • Patients maybe agitated and moving a lot in bed	• Intermittent positive pressure breathing (IPPB), noninvasive ventilation (NIV) may be useful to augment vital expansion • Breath stacking, manual assisted cough or MIE can all be used prophylactically • In the absence of appropriate supported seating, may need to use extra pillows or specialist equipment to aid posture
Increased work of breathing	• From muscle weakness or fatigue?	• Positioning • IPPB and NIV may be helpful
Respiratory failure	• Watch out for fatigue, call for help early!	• IPPB and NIV • An early call to critical care is always appropriate if the patient has not reached their ceiling of care
Immobility	• Manage by good and regular repositioning • Appropriate seating can help, this can be difficult in acute patients because of lack of seating, agitation and drains etc	• If no contraindications are present alternate side lying with trunk rotations ± manual techniques can mobilise secretions

Continued

TABLE 14.5	PATIENT PROBLEMS AND PHYSIOTHERAPY INTERVENTIONS—cont'd	
PROBLEM	CONSIDER	PHYSIOTHERAPY INTERVENTIONS
Fear/ anxiety/ agitation	• Patients can be cognitively affected. Ideally agitated patients will have management strategies in place. If not, liaise with the multidisciplinary team for your own safety • Fear and anxiety affect these patients. Empathy and understanding are essential, balanced against a need to explain the consequences of refusing treatment	• Remain calm and seek guidance • Ask the nursing staff to assist you or simply be present

SUMMARY

Good assessment identifies subtle changes in these patient's respiratory status. Physiotherapy is key because of their high risk of respiratory deterioration.

Think about positioning first; this can make patients feel more comfortable, as well as improve ventilation.

Fear and anxiety are common, build a rapport with your patient, they know what works for them so listen!

References and further reading

Brain Trauma Foundation Guidelines, 2016. Accessed at https://braintrauma.org/upload s/07/04/Guidelines_for_the_Management_of_Severe_Traumatic.97250__2_.pdf.

Chin, L.S., 2018. Spinal cord injuries. Accessed at: https://emedicine.medscape.com/arti cle/793582-clinical.

Glasgow Coma Scale. Accessed at https://www.glasgowcomascale.org/

Lennon, S., Ramdharry, G., Verheyden, G., 2018. Physical Management for Neurological Conditions, fourth ed. Elsevier, London.

van Aswegen, H., Morrow, B., 2015. Cardiopulmonary Physiotherapy in Trauma: An Evidence-Based Approach. Imperial College Press, London.

CHAPTER 15

WORKING ON THE CARDIOTHORACIC UNIT

Leanne McCarthy

INTRODUCTION

Physiotherapy is an important element of care for patients on the cardiothoracic unit, which includes those having cardiothoracic surgery, with cardiothoracic trauma or those with a cardiology issue.

AIMS

By the end of this chapter you should:

- Understand different cardiothoracic surgery procedures and common incisions
- Understand the assessment and treatment of patients following:
  - Cardiac and thoracic surgery
  - Cardiothoracic trauma
  - Cardiology issues
- Recognise common patient problems and be able to modify clinical interventions

THE ENVIRONMENT

In the cardiothoracic unit, patients are often monitored with many invasive lines, for example, central and arterial lines and cardiac monitoring (pulse index contour continuous cardiac output) all linked to alarms. Postoperative patients may also have other attachments, including pacing boxes, chest drains and epidural or epipleural catheters. Although some of this may be new, remember the nursing staff are on hand to help if you are unsure of anything.

THE POPULATION

Cardiac Surgery

Cardiac surgery is any surgical procedure carried out on the heart or great vessels. Common procedures and incisions are summarised in Table 15.1 and Appendix 3. Although many procedures can now be carried out using minimally invasive techniques.

This surgery usually requires cardiopulmonary bypass, however, 'off pump' surgery is becoming more common for some of their coronary artery bypass graft (CABG) procedures, as evidence shows it can reduce postoperative complications.

Knowing the surgical techniques and procedure are important details, as they affect your assessment and management of the patient, for example, median sternotomy or thoracotomy causes decreased lung capacities, increasing likelihood of postoperative pulmonary complications (PPC).

Thoracic Surgery

Thoracic surgery is normally for resection of cancerous lung tissue (lobectomy, pneumonectomy, wedge resection), management of a recurrent pleural problems (decortication, pleurectomy, pleurodesis), removal of bullae (or lung volume reduction surgery) or to repair a chest wall deformity.

TABLE 15.1 CARDIAC SURGERY

TYPE OF INCISION	EXAMPLES OF COMMON PROCEDURES
Median Sternotomy	Coronary artery bypass graft (CABG) Valve repair or replacement Aortic surgery, including repair of dissections or aneurysms Removal of thymoma Heart/lung transplantation
Minimally Invasive	Valve repair or replacement endoscopically or via anterior right thoracotomy Endoscopic CABG Minimally invasive direct coronary artery bypass grafting Transcatheter aortic valve implantation Cardiac surgery via hemisternotomy
Thoracotomy	Aortic surgery

The surgical incision will depend on the nature and extent of the surgery. Most procedures are now carried out using video-assisted thoracic surgery (VATs), however, a posterolateral thoracotomy may also be required. VATs is minimally invasive, which reduces the impact on respiratory function, limits the amount of trauma, shortens hospital stay, produces less postoperative pain and has less impact on postoperative shoulder movements than open surgery and faster return to activity (Socci & Martin-Ucar, 2016).

Cardiothoracic Trauma

Cardiothoracic trauma patients can have isolated thoracic trauma, but often have additional trauma injuries. These patients may have significant pulmonary compromise from injuries which include:

- Rib fractures (including flail segment)
- Stab injuries
- Lung contusions and/or haematoma
- Pneumothorax/haemothorax

Many are managed conservatively but some patients will require interventions, such as insertion of an intercostal chest drain or surgical stabilisation of a flail segment

Cardiology

Respiratory physiotherapy is rarely indicated in acute cardiology patients, but they are prone to developing associated problems after, particularly if they are immobile. Development of a hospital acquired pneumonia or infected pulmonary oedema are possibilities (see Chapter 11 Medical chapter).

Conditions include:

- Myocardial infarction
- Congestive cardiac failure
- Coronary artery disease
- Arrhythmias

ASSESSING THE CARDIOTHORACIC PATIENT

Preoperative status is important, as it may predispose patients to a higher risk of PPC (see Surgery Chapter 10).

These patients often have chronic lung disease, as smoking is a common risk factor, and a higher risk of respiratory infection/compromise,

PPCs, prolonged respiratory support, longer intensive care stay and increased mortality.

Specialist Equipment
In specialist centres, you will see equipment, including extracorporeal membrane oxygenation and ventricular assist devices. Follow your trust guidance for managing these patients and ensure your competence with preparation and training. Specific considerations around monitoring and attachments are discussed later. Key considerations for each patient group are summarised in Table 15.2.

Analgesia
Postoperative pain is expected, however, the patient needs appropriate analgesia for assessment and treatment. Multidisciplinary team (MDT) considerations will ensure effective analgesia and monitoring for side effects.

Neurological
Patients undergoing cardiac surgery may have sustained a neurological deficit which may not be evident clinically. The most common cause is cerebral hypoperfusion, following low perfusion pressures, embolic occlusion of vessels, hypothermia and hypoxaemia. These may manifest as confusion, seizures or weakness and affect postoperative care.

Time on Bypass Machine
Cardiopulmonary bypass involves the heart being stopped and the circulating blood being removed, filtered and oxygenated outside the body, before being returned to the body. During bypass, the lungs are collapsed. This results in increased intra- and extravascular fluid, increased pulmonary vascular resistance, decreased lung compliance, decreased functional residual capacity, producing atelectasis and intrapulmonary shunting.

Intraaortic Balloon Pump
The intraaortic balloon pump (IABP) supports blood pressure by increasing cardiac output by as much as 40%, reducing myocardial workload and improving coronary artery blood flow. Patients with an IABP in situ will be on strict bed rest, hip flexion is limited to 30 degrees to avoid displacement. Thus you must take care with positioning and manual techniques and bagging may be restricted. Follow your trust guidelines.

TABLE 15.2 ASSESSMENT CONSIDERATIONS

	CARDIAC SURGERY	THORACIC SURGERY	CARDIOTHORACIC TRAUMA	CARDIOLOGY
Central Nervous System	Effective analgesia Neurological status	Effective analgesia Neurological status	Effective analgesia	Neurological status
Cardiovascular	External Pacemaker dependency Intraaortic balloon pump Heart rate/rhythm Inotrope dependency	Effects of analgesia for example, Epidural/epipleural	Effects of analgesia for example, epidural/epipleural	Cardiac function
Respiratory	Chest drains CXR Arterial blood gases (ABGs) Respiratory rate/pattern Oxygen requirement	Chest drains ± suction Chest x-ray (CXR) Thoracic expansion Respiratory rate/pattern Oxygen requirement	Chest drains ± suction CXR Thoracic expansion Respiratory rate / pattern Oxygen requirement	CXR Respiratory rate / pattern Oxygen requirement
Renal	Renal insult affecting respiratory status			
Biochemistry	Inflammatory markers ABGs	Histology result (if appropriate) Inflammatory markers	Inflammatory markers	
Be aware of…	Invasive monitoring Time on bypass		Additional injuries, for example, head injury Or other fractures	Ongoing medical plan, e.g., revascularisation, angioplasty, pharmacological management May have rib fractures from cardiopulmonary resuscitation efforts

Arrhythmias/Changes in Heart Rate

Cardiac surgery patients commonly develop arrhythmias postoperatively because of changes in automaticity and conduction. Arrhythmias, which affect cardiac output, include atrial fibrillation and atrial flutter, ventricular and supraventricular tachycardia, ventricular ectopics, bradycardia and some heart blocks. These may limit or affect treatment, discuss with the MDT before making treatment decisions.

Inotropes

Cardiac output can be reduced postoperatively and inotropes may be used to increase blood pressure. Some interventions reduce cardiac output, including positive pressure and mobilisation, so discuss with the MDT, to determine any scope to increase pharmacological support if required. Blood pressure may be deliberately kept within certain limits to protect the surgical site.

Pacing

Intraoperatively pacing wires are placed on the myocardium, with leads externally connected to a pacing box, as patients are very prone to arrhythmias and intrinsic pacing problems. It is important to note if the patient is dependent on this pacing and be very aware of the delicate wires that enter through the chest when mobilising the patient. When pacing wires are removed, patients should not mobilise immediately—check your trust guidance.

Respiratory

Patients in the cardiothoracic unit have the same respiratory monitoring as other areas, they may be ventilated for a short period immediately postoperative.

Intercostal Chest Drains

An air leak is the escape of air into the pleura after cardiothoracic surgery and manifests as bubbling on an underwater seal or a digital reading on digital chest drains. Postoperatively, chest drains are routinely positioned to drain residual fluid/air, restore normal negative pleural pressure and facilitate lung reexpansion. Removal usually occurs when there is no fluid draining and no visible air leak. A chest x-ray (CXR) after drain removal is required to ensure there is no pneumothorax.

Low-pressure thoracic suction may be applied to the chest drain to assist drainage. In most instances this can be disconnected for mobilisation, as it is thought that exercise and resulting bigger lung volumes facilitate drainage. Check your trust policy and confirm with ward staff before taking a patient off suction. Portable digital chest drain systems allow patients to mobilise without disconnecting suction.

The escape of air into subcutaneous tissues is surgical emphysema and signifies the need to rule out a pneumothorax. Surgical emphysema is palpable under the skin, dependent on its severity (think snap, crackle and pop!) and identified on CXR as black areas (air) in soft tissue shadows.

Be aware—pneumothorax can occur after chest drain removal, which will affect treatment choices. Always check CXR, after drain removal, before using positive pressure devices. Any changes in auscultation after chest drain removal should be raised with the medical team.

Renal

The kidneys can incur acute injury following surgery and reduced cardiac output. This presents as reduce urine output and increasing fluid overload. This affects the respiratory status, increasing the likelihood of pulmonary oedema and pleural effusions. Aortic aneurysm repairs can also damage the kidneys by reducing the blood supply via the renal artery depending on the aneurysm position.

Clinical reasoning

Cardiothoracic patients are susceptible to PPCs in the same way as other surgical patients with additional risk from:
- Time on bypass machine (cardiac patients)
- Direct injury to lungs (thoracic or trauma patients)
- Pain from chest drains

Other common complications – Table 15.3

Left lower lobe collapse is common and lung volumes can take up to 2 weeks to return to normal after cardiothoracic surgery. Up to 40% of patients undergoing cardiac surgery develop pleural effusions. Internal mammary artery (IMA) harvesting is associated with a higher rate of ipsilateral pleural effusions (Chikwe et al., 2013).

Permanent or temporary damage or paresis to either phrenic nerve may occur when opening the chest, harvesting the IMA, creating a window in the pleura or using topical cooling. This causes the related hemidiaphragm to rise and may look like lung collapse.

TABLE 15.3 COMMON COMPLICATIONS POSTCARDIAC SURGERY

PROBLEM	CAUSE	MEDICAL MANAGEMENT	PHYSIOTHERAPY CONSIDERATIONS
Neurological deficit	Intraoperative hypoxia Cerebral ischaemia	May require prolonged ventilation manage coagulation	Increased risk of aspiration and respiratory compromise
Pain	Operative procedure Incision site Chest drains (heightened by anxiety)	Analgesia	Upper limb movement and thoracic expansion can help ease musculoskeletal stiffness Discuss with MDT regarding timing and effectiveness of analgesia
Renal impairment	Renal hypoperfusion perioperatively	Fluid management, diuretics haemofiltration	Care with haemofiltration lines Be aware of associated hypotension Respiratory compromise from fluid overload
Hypotension	Cardiac failure Hypovolaemia	Inotropic support Fluid resuscitation IABP	Caution with positive pressure (IPPB, CPAP, MHI) and mobilisation
Hypertension	Pain and agitation Disruption to patient's normal drug regime	Nitrates or beta-blockers	May be aggravated with exercise and inadequate analgesia May limit mobilisation

Continued

TABLE 15.3 COMMON COMPLICATIONS POSTCARDIAC SURGERY—cont'd

PROBLEM	CAUSE	MEDICAL MANAGEMENT	PHYSIOTHERAPY CONSIDERATIONS
Arrhythmias/ Heart Block	Biochemical derangement (e.g., hypokalaemia), AV bruising intraoperatively, Electrical pathway disturbance	Amiodarone, Digoxin, pacing, cardioversion	Do not mobilise if HR>120 bpm or BP compromised Patient may be reliant on external cardiac pacing If in heart block, caution with mobilisation
Cardiac tamponade	Collection of fluid inside the pericardium can lead to cardiac arrest	Immediate surgical intervention	Physiotherapy contraindicated
Myocardial Infarction	Inadequate myocardial perfusion	GTN infusion, ECG monitoring Troponin levels	Follow trust guidance on mobilisation
Sternal wound infection (can lead to mediastinitis)	Infection	Antibiotics, vac-pump	Extra sternal precautions will apply If sternum fails to unite will alter respiratory mechanics and impede effective cough
Pleural effusion	Premature removal of chest drains Poor positioning of chest drains Low serum protein, poor nutritional status Persistent bleeding	Insertion/ repositioning of chest drain	Chest drain precautions Oxygen therapy

TABLE 15.3	COMMON COMPLICATIONS POSTCARDIAC SURGERY—cont'd		
PROBLEM	**CAUSE**	**MEDICAL MANAGEMENT**	**PHYSIOTHERAPY CONSIDERATIONS**
Pulmonary oedema	Fluid overload Deranged fluid balance	Diuresis CPAP	Prolonged episodes can lead to infective changes, which may need physiotherapy intervention
Pneumothorax	Failure of pleura to adhere	Chest drain insertion (may be conservatively managed if pneumothorax small)	Expansion exercises Positive pressure treatments often contraindicated
Lobe collapse	General anaesthetic Sputum plugging Pain and insufficient respiratory effort	Oxygen therapy If ventilated can manipulate settings, for example, increase peep	See Interventions Table 15.5
Sputum retention Chest infection	Impaired cough Sputum retention	Antibiotics	See Interventions Table 15.5
Hypoxaemia	Impaired gaseous exchange	Depends on cause	Ensure adequate oxygenation throughout treatment

AV, Atrioventricular; *BP,* blood pressure; *CPAP,* continuous positive airway pressure; *ECG,* electrocardiogram; *GTN,* glyceryl trinitrate; *HR,* heart rate; *IABP,* intraaortic balloon pump; *IPPB,* intermittent positive pressure breathing; *MDT,* multidisciplinary team; *MHI,* manual hyperinflation.

Cardiothoracic Trauma

Physiotherapy may be indicated for patients with rib fractures who develop respiratory compromise or sputum retention. Patients with lung contusions often present with very bloody, pluggy sputum. Associated problems of cardiothoracic trauma include pain, reduced thoracic expansion, altered breathing pattern, impaired cough, potential for chest infection/sputum retention and hypoxaemia.

TABLE 15.4 COMMON COMPLICATIONS AFTER THORACIC SURGERY

PROBLEM	CAUSE	MEDICAL MANAGEMENT	PHYSIOTHERAPY CONSIDERATIONS
Pain	Incision site Operative procedure and position Chest drain	Analgesia Epidural/ epipleural	Optimise analgesia pretreatment With epidural, check lower limb function and blood pressure before mobilisation Upper limb and thoracic exercises in comfortable range can help if pain exacerbated by anxiety
Persistent air leak in drain	Failure of pleural adhesion	Suction applied to intercostal drain	Mobilisation Consider exercise bike
Surgical emphysema	Air leak into subcutaneous space on insertion or removal of chest drain	Oxygen therapy If severe, small superficial skin incisions can be made to release the air	Auscultation can be difficult Check chest x-ray Caution with positive pressure devices
Lung collapse	Sputum plugging, failure of lung to reexpand postintraoperative deflation Pain, insufficient respiratory effort	Depends on cause Analgesia bronchoscopy if severe sputum plugging	See Interventions Table 15.5
Sputum retention	General anaesthetic – impaired mucociliary clearance Impaired cough	Nebulisers Systemic hydration Humidified oxygen	Monitor inflammatory markers See Interventions Table 15.5
Hypoxaemia	Impaired gas exchange	Depends on cause	Optimise oxygen therapy
Musculoskeletal dysfunction	Incision site Operative position	Analgesia if pain related	May limit thoracic expansion/shoulder movement Outpatient follow-up as needed

Cardiology Patients

Patient's cardiac function may affect their respiratory system, that is, pulmonary oedema and pleural effusion. Consult the medical team to clarify.

Clinical interventions

Cardiothoracic Surgery

Management dictated by identification of the cause (see Table 15.5). These patients can deteriorate very quickly, particularly following thoracic surgery. There is little reliable evidence supporting prophylactic respiratory physiotherapy however, deep breathing, expectoration and mobilisation are usually encouraged.

The value of mobilisation after cardiothoracic surgery is well established (Westerdahl, 2015) and all postoperative patients should follow a progressive mobilisation programme from day 1.

In at-risk patients, numerous interventions are effective in promoting airway clearance for example, upright positioning, active cycle of breathing technique and ambulation (Pasquina et al., 2003). There is no evidence for incentive spirometry. More recently, positive expiratory pressure (Urell et al., 2011) and inspiratory muscle training (Mans et al., 2015) have been investigated but these are not widely used yet.

CARDIOTHORACIC TRAUMA

Patients with cardiothoracic trauma benefit from nebulisers and humidification to facilitate sputum clearance. Mobilisation should be encouraged. Care should be taken with manual techniques (dependent on injuries). A chest x-ray should be taken before any positive pressure techniques because of possible pneumothorax.

Cardiology Patients

Cardiology patients presenting with respiratory compromise should be encouraged to mobilise. Consider cardiovascular (CVS) instability, electrocardiogram changes and any assist devices e.g. IABP, before intervention. Ensure adequate oxygenation throughout to prevent further CVS stress. Manual techniques are avoided if the patient has rib fractures after cardiopulmonary resuscitation.

Continuous positive airway pressure could be considered for pulmonary oedema.

Cardiac Rehabilitation

Cardiac rehabilitation has shown significant benefits for short- and long-term recovery after cardiac surgery or acute cardiac event. Identify your local service provision and referrals and actively encourage patients to attend.

TABLE 15.5	INTERVENTIONS FOR COMMON PROBLEMS IN CARDIOTHORACIC SURGICAL PATIENTS (SEE CHAPTER 9 TREATMENTS)
PROBLEM AND PRESENTATION	**PHYSIOTHERAPY MANAGEMENT**

Lung collapse Unilateral or bilateral volume loss on chest x-ray Hypoxaemia Increased work of breathing Poor tidal volume Reduced BS on auscultation Reduced thoracic expansion	• Progressive mobilisation
	  • Use ambulatory oxygen in hypoxaemic patients
	  • May be limited to bedside if on strict wall suction
	  • Consider alternatives (e.g., exercise bike where appropriate)
	
	IPPB : (may be through manual insufflation/exsufflation [MI:E] devices)
	• May have only transient effect—consider in combination with CPAP
	• Ensure flow is high enough to meet demand, then reduced as patient settles
	• Check x-ray before to rule out pneumothorax
	• Get surgeon approval before intervention because of anastomosis
	
	CPAP
	• Ensure adequate PEEP—larger patients or those with significant collapse will need a PEEP of 10 cmH$_2$O
	• Ensure flow meets demand—consider size of patient and inspiratory demand
	• If recent drain removal, check x-ray before use
	
	Lower thoracic expansion exercises
	• Less effective than mobilisation, but useful if mobilisation contraindicated
	• Use in combination with appropriate positioning
	• Try end inspiratory hold and/or sniff

PROBLEM AND PRESENTATION	PHYSIOTHERAPY MANAGEMENT
Sputum retention Added sounds on auscultation (crackles, wheezes) Increased work of breathing Increased respiratory rate Poor tidal volume Palpable fremitus Wet, weak cough Hypoxaemia Respiratory fatigue Possible raised inflammatory markers	Progressive mobilisation if poor tidal volume is the cause **IPPB** • Intersperse with sputum clearance • Use manual techniques in conjunction if able • Get surgeon approval before intervention because of anastomosis **Manual techniques** • Ensure adequate analgesia • Avoid vibs/shaking if sternum unstable • Avoid surgical wound and chest drains **Positioning** • Use with above techniques • Consider cardiovascular (CVS) status and lines/drains • Avoid side lying in pneumonectomy patients. This increases risk of stump break down and development of bronchopleural fistula **Manual hyperinflation (if intubated)** • If manual techniques alone prove ineffective and CVS will tolerate • Use in conjunction with manual techniques and positioning • Get surgeon approval before intervention because of anastomosis **Suction** • Endotracheal for intubated patients • Nasopharyngeal (NP): check clotting especially if patient is on haemofiltration and heparinised • Use NP airway for repeated suctioning to prevent trauma **Supported cough** • Cough-locks or support towels can be used • Reassure patient that sternum is well wired **MI:E** • Ensure weak cough is not caused by insufficient analgesia • Check x-ray to rule out pneumothorax • Not routinely used in thoracic surgery patients

BS, breath sounds; *CPAP*, continuous positive airway pressure; *IPPB*, intermittent positive pressure breathing; *PEEP*, positive end expiratory pressure.

Summary

- You are a vital part of the cardiothoracic unit.
- Remember, functional rehabilitation and secondary prevention of further occurrences, for example, cardiac rehabilitation are important.

References

Chikwe, J., et al., 2013. Cardiothoracic Surgery, 2nd ed. Oxford University Press, Oxford.

Mans, C.M., Reeve, J.C., Elkins, M.R., 2015. Postoperative outcomes following preoperative inspiratory muscle training in patients undergoing cardiothoracic or upper abdominal surgery: a systematic review and meta analysis. Clin. Rehabil. 29 (5), 426–438.

Pasquina, P., et al., 2003. Prophylactic respiratory physiotherapy after cardiac surgery: systematic review. BMJ. 327, 1379–1385.

Socci, L., Martin-Ucar, A.E., 2016. Access to the chest cavity: Safeguards and Pitfalls. In: Scarci, M., et al. (Eds.), Core Topics in Thoracic Surgery. Cambridge university press.

Urell, C., et al., 2011. et al. Deep breathing exercises with positive expiratory pressure at a higher rate improve oxygenation in the early period after cardiac surgery a randomised controlled trial. Eur. J. Cardiothorac. Surg. 40 (1), 162–167.

Westerdahl, E., 2015. Optimal technique for deep breathing exercises after cardiac surgery. Minerva Anestesiol. 81, 678–683.

CHAPTER 16

PAEDIATRIC WARDS

Claire Hepworth

INTRODUCTION AND ENVIRONMENT

Paediatric wards hold a wide variety of patients, including, medical, surgical, neurological, neuromuscular and oncology. You will be part of a multidisciplinary team (MDT), which works together holistically to improve outcomes. Although every child's presentation is unique, the core respiratory assessment remains the same.

AIMS
By the end of this chapter you should be able to:
- Review a paediatric respiratory assessment
- Identify and clinically reason a problem list
- Discuss the physiotherapy management for these problems
- Identify the effectiveness of treatment techniques
- Identify guidelines for working with children

THE POPULATION

Assessment
Consent should be gained before assessing the patient, in children this is different (see Chapter 2 Assessment). Assessment is a holistic overview of the body systems, but remember they interconnect, for example, pyrexia can cause tachypnoea because of increased metabolic demand, sepsis will cause respiratory distress.

Subjective assessment is obtained from medical notes, nursing handover and information from the patient and parent. Establishing a good rapport with the child, parents and families, explaining your assessment findings and proposed treatment, helps their understanding, cooperation and follow-on care.

Your objective assessment confirms the subjective information.

TABLE 16.1   PAEDIATRIC RESPIRATORY ASSESSMENT

Respiratory

Monitor	Considerations
Patency of airway	• Can the child maintain their own airway? • If not, call the resus team, they need urgent nasopharyngeal/oropharyngeal airway or endotracheal tube intubation.
Oxygen requirement and saturations	• How stable is the patient? • If they desaturate, is there scope to increase their oxygen? • Is it humidified? • Check the trace from the oxygenation saturation probe does it reflect a good contact with the finger/ear.
Work of breathing (WOB): respiratory rate, nasal flare, tracheal tug, subcostal/intercostal/sternal recession, expiratory grunt, accessory muscle use	• Increased WOB can lead to fatigue, which may mean the child is unable to sustain their ventilation. • No increased WOB when there should be, indicates exhaustion and imminent respiratory arrest.
Stridor	• Upper respiratory tract obstruction. Physiotherapy is contraindicated. • Manage by jaw thrust manoeuvre and call for help.
Chest expansion	• Is it symmetrical?
Breathing pattern	• NOTE: handling can change the breathing pattern. • Apical or diaphragmatic—related to patient's age. • Signs of hypoventilation? • Prolonged expiration indicating bronchospasm.
Palpable or audible secs	• Suggestive of upper respiratory tract secretions.
Auscultation findings	• Ensure all areas are listened to. • Are there breath sounds throughout? • Are there added sounds?

Cardiovascular

Monitor	Considerations

TABLE 16.1 PAEDIATRIC RESPIRATORY ASSESSMENT—cont'd

Heart rate	• Any medicine induced changes? • Tachycardia—increased WOB, pain, fever • Bradycardia—secretion retention, sedatives • Arrhythmias—is the patient cardiovascularly stable?
Mucous membranes/colour	• Dry—dehydration • Pale—anaemia, poor perfusion.
Capillary refill	• Performed over the manubriosternum in children (see Chapter 3)
Temperature	• Febrile convulsion?
Blood Pressure	• Hypotension leads to poor perfusion

Central nervous system

Monitor	Considerations
Responsiveness	• Brain perfusion and oxygenation
Seizures	• Do not perform physiotherapy during seizure
Preexisting pathology	• Altered tone affecting handling/positioning/increased stridor

Renal/gastrointestinal

Monitor	Considerations
Abdominal distention	• Splints the diaphragm, reduced lung volumes, increased WOB, atelectasis because of compression
Dehydration	• Increased viscosity of secretions
Fluid overload	• Potential pulmonary oedema

Abnormal bleeding/ coagulation

Monitor	Considerations
Platelet/coagulation markers	• Identify any cautions/contraindications to treatments for example, platelet count <50, consider risk vs. benefit to percussion, expiratory vibrations and nasopharyngeal suction • Risk of pulmonary haemorrhage?
Actively bleeding from attachments	• Clinical signs of bruising/petechiae/fresh blood around lines/drains • Consider positioning, saline nebulisers, ACBT, gentle mobilisation before other physiotherapy treatments

Continued

TABLE 16.1 PAEDIATRIC RESPIRATORY ASSESSMENT—cont'd

Musculoskeletal

Monitor	Considerations
Bone density problems for example, osteoporosis Rib/spinal fractures	• Identify risk vs. benefit of percussion, expiratory vibrations and nasopharyngeal suction

Other

Monitor	Considerations
Infection markers	• Where is the source of the infection?
X-ray/CT scan/USS	• Identify acute and chronic respiratory problems
Blood gases	• Interpret blood gas if available
Feeding	• Poor feeding may be caused by increased WOB
Sputum results	• Bacterial or viral infection?

ACBT, Active cycle of breathing technique; *CT*, computed tomography; *USS*, ultrasound scan.

Assessment starts from the moment you can see the patient, noting their position and signs of respiratory distress (for normal values and paediatrics specifics, see Chapter 3). Note the patient's medication, particularly respiratory drugs for example, mucolytics (saline/hypertonic saline nebulisers), antimuscarinics (hyoscine/glycopyrrolate), antibiotics, and potential sedatives. Ensure you identify cautions/contraindications to treatment.

But if you walk into a child's room and they have low oxygen saturations (<92%), not normal for them, address this before conducting the assessment. Sustained low saturations causes hypoxic tissue damage and remember, there is a delay in oxygenation saturations, reflecting what is happening to the child.

Children deteriorate more quickly than adults, ensure you are fully prepared with any equipment that may be required, know where resuscitation equipment is, how to contact the resuscitation team and what to do before their arrival.

CLINICAL REASONING/TREATMENT

Identify a problem list with possible explanations, key abnormal markers and consider what treatments are indicated or not. Always reassess to evaluate your treatment effectiveness and if ineffective consider alternatives including reassessing problem list.

MEDICAL PATIENTS

TABLE 16.2	RESPIRATORY PROBLEMS, DIAGNOSTIC FINDINGS AND POTENTIAL PHYSIOTHERAPY MANAGEMENT
Pneumonia/Consolidation: Acute and resolving	
Overview	• **Acute:** Consolidated 'dense' area of inflammatory exudate and pus in the alveoli • **Resolving:** Exudate is broken down by enzymes and either remains dry and drains via lymphatic system or presents as retained secretions
History	• **Acute:** Pyrexia, breathlessness, increased work of breathing (WOB), dry cough, reduced oxygen saturations • **Resolving:** As earlier, except may have a wet cough
Expansion	• Can affect expansion if large/multilobar
Auscultation	• **Acute:** Bronchial breath sounds • **Resolving:** Reduced breath sounds or crackles particularly on inspiration.
Percussion note	• Dull
Chest x-ray (CXR)	• White, dense area occupying partial/complete lobes, but can also be 'patchy white' • No fissure shift. No tracheal/mediastinal shift • No volume loss • Blurring of hemidiaphragm if present in lower zone • Potential air bronchogram
Medical management	• IV antibiotics, IV fluids, oxygen, supportive care

Continued

TABLE 16.2	RESPIRATORY PROBLEMS, DIAGNOSTIC FINDINGS AND POTENTIAL PHYSIOTHERAPY MANAGEMENT—cont'd
Physiotherapy management	**Acute:** • No manual chest therapy techniques • Position for ventilation/perfusion ($\dot{V}/\dot{Q}$) matching to optimise good lung if in respiratory distress • Mobility/upper limb exercises/ play/posture/regular repositioning • Lung expansion exercises—ACBT, blowing games, incentive spirometry **Resolving:** • As earlier, but no need for positioning for $\dot{V}/\dot{Q}$ matching • Manual chest therapy may be indicated • Consider if PEP and mucolytics are necessary
Retained secretions with or without volume loss	
Overview	• Secretions in the lower respiratory tract because of infection, exacerbation of respiratory condition, pain, weak cough or impaired mucociliary escalator
History	• Productive cough can occur in the absence of infection • Breathlessness, increased WOB, reduced oxygen saturations
Expansion	• Expansion reduced on affected lung
Auscultation	• Reduced breath sounds • Crackles on auscultation
Percussion note	• Dull
CXR	• White, dense area often occupying partial/complete lobes • Fissure shift and 'sail sign' if in lower lobe • Tracheal/mediastinal shift towards the collapse • Volume loss on affected side (raised hemidiaphragm, rib crowding) • Blurring of hemidiaphragm if present in lower zone
Medical management	• Supportive care • Humidification—oxygen (ideally heated), mucolytics • If infection—antibiotics
Physiotherapy management	• Same as resolving consolidation

TABLE 16.2	RESPIRATORY PROBLEMS, DIAGNOSTIC FINDINGS AND POTENTIAL PHYSIOTHERAPY MANAGEMENT—cont'd

Pleural effusion and empyema

Overview	**Pleural effusion:** • Excess fluid in the pleural space • Can develop with pneumonia or postsurgery **Empyema:** • Infected pleural effusion and fluid is thick and loculated **Either pleural effusion or empyema:** • Can compress the underlying lung—collapse • Potential underlying consolidation
History	• Pain, pyrexia, breathlessness, dry cough, increased WOB, reduced oxygen saturations
Expansion	• Usually normal
Auscultation	• Absent breath sounds or reduced breath sounds when resolving
Percussion note	• Dull
CXR	**Pleural effusion:** • White area that is gravity dependent (check position x-ray was taken in) • Fluid line at bottom of lung in upright x-ray and fluid 'cap' at top of lung • Hazy white area over whole lung in supine position with blunted costophrenic angle **Empyema:** • Dense white area that is not specific to lobes • Not dependent on x-ray position **Pleural effusion or empyema:** Diagnosed via ultrasound scan • No mediastinal shift unless very large (away from side of effusion) • No volume loss • Blurring of hemidiaphragm if in lower zone

Continued

TABLE 16.2	RESPIRATORY PROBLEMS, DIAGNOSTIC FINDINGS AND POTENTIAL PHYSIOTHERAPY MANAGEMENT—cont'd
Medical management	**Pleural effusion:** • Chest drain ± low-grade suction **Empyema:** • Chest drain ± low-grade suction and intrapleural fibrinolytic agents, for example, urokinase inserted into chest drain and temporarily clamped • If unsuccessful, thoracocentesis, pleurodesis, lung resection and decortication may be considered **Pleural effusion and empyema:** • Antibiotics if infective, oxygen, pain relief, supportive care
Physiotherapy management	**Pleural effusion and empyema:** • Physiotherapy will not directly affect pleural effusion or empyema • Physiotherapy indicated to maintain/improve lung expansion under the affected pleura • Physiotherapy includes lung expansion exercises for example, mobilisation, upper limb exercises, postural exercises, ACBT, incentive spirometry possibly, regular repositioning and supported cough **Empyema:** • Physiotherapy intervention maximised if used when intrapleural fibrinolytic agents clamped in drain
Pneumothorax	
Overview	• Collection of air in the pleural space • Can be spontaneous or traumatic or caused by underlying lung pathology • If large needs urgent treatment
History	• Can occur suddenly, pain, breathlessness, reduced oxygen saturations
Expansion	• Reduced on affected side
Auscultation	• Absent breath sounds on affected side
Percussion note	• Hyperresonant
CXR	• Black, hyperinflated, no lung markings on affected side • Visible visceral pleural edge (thin, sharp white line) • Mediastinal shift only if tension pneumothorax
Medical management	• Chest drain, oxygen, pain relief, supportive care

TABLE 16.2	RESPIRATORY PROBLEMS, DIAGNOSTIC FINDINGS AND POTENTIAL PHYSIOTHERAPY MANAGEMENT—cont'd
Physiotherapy management	• Physiotherapy will not directly affect the pneumothorax • Physiotherapy may improve underlying lung collapse • Lung expansion exercises for example, mobilisation, upper limb and postural exercises, regular repositioning and ACBT. Remember to keep chest drain below level of insertion • No positive pressure devices if undrained pneumothorax and with care with drained pneumothorax

Pulmonary oedema

Overview	• Fluid accumulation in the alveoli and between the alveoli and capillaries
History	• Breathlessness—particularly when lying down (orthopnoea), reduced oxygen saturations, sweating, pain, increased WOB, pink frothy secretions
Expansion	• Normal
Auscultation	• Fine end inspiratory crackles, position dependent
Percussion note	• Normal or dull
CXR	• White perihilar haze 'cotton wool appearance' • Thickening of bronchial walls • Increased cardiac size • Air bronchograms? • Position dependent
Medical management	• Oxygen, diuretics, supportive care for ventilation and cardiac support
Physiotherapy management	• Physiotherapy will not affect pulmonary oedema • Oedema cleared by suction will reaccumulate • Treat other underlying respiratory problems • Optimise $\dot{V}/\dot{Q}$

ACBT, Active cycle of breathing technique; *IV*, intravenous; *PEP*, positive end expiratory pressure. *V/P*, ventilation/perfusion.

TIPS FOR ASSESSMENT AND TREATMENT

• More than one problem can occur in the same lung, at the same time, for example, patches of collapse and consolidation. Use your clinical reasoning, try a treatment, reassess and revaluate what the main problem is.

- When treating a patient in respiratory distress, with a collapsed lung, the affected lung should be uppermost, however, this can increase WOB, so increase oxygenation during physiotherapy. If unable to tolerate this position, consider prone with monitoring.
- Use toys, games and distraction techniques for treatment. Never hold a child down, unless they are going to hurt themselves.
- A blocked nose in an infant can cause respiratory distress. Consider clearing with saline nose drops or nasopharyngeal suction—or simply a tissue.
- Repeated infections can cause bronchiectasis therefore ensure treatments are effective while in hospital and consider whether parents/carers should to be trained to deliver physiotherapy at home.
- Always consider giving patients, families and nursing staff advice to continue interventions between physiotherapy sessions to optimise outcomes for example, for a patient with left lower lobe collapse you may advice regular repositioning, including high right side lying, saline/hypertonic saline nebulisers and nasopharyngeal suction as indicated.
- Oxygen over 2 L/min should be humidified, otherwise it can dry the airways and secretions.

CYSTIC FIBROSIS/BRONCHIECTASIS/PRIMARY CILIARY DYSKINESIA/IMMUNE DEFICIENCY/CHRONIC LUNG DISEASE

These patients have preexisting pathology that predisposes them to chest infections. They require an individualised chest physiotherapy management plan for airway clearance and exercise. Hospital admissions are an opportunity to review management plans, participation in those plans and exercise tolerance. This often includes positioning, manual chest techniques, positive end expiratory pressure (PEP) and oscillating-PEP adjuncts, mucolytics and exercise. Computed tomography reports and chest x-rays can guide targeted physiotherapy treatment, such as saline nasal irrigation, review of posture/musculoskeletal problems and inspiratory muscle training. Autogenic drainage can be considered if the patient is sufficiently motivated to learn the technique. Postural drainage positions can be used in some children but be aware a head down position may cause aspiration and should only be used if benefits out way the risk. Encourage children to be independent with airway clearance techniques, but when admitted with acute exacerbation or they are tired, manual chest physiotherapy should be considered.

There are comprehensive guidelines for physiotherapy management:

- British Thoracic Society (BTS) guidelines for non-cystic fibrosis bronchiectasis (2010).
- National Institute for Care and Health Excellence guidelines in cystic fibrosis (2017).

Standards of Care and Good Clinical Practice for the Physiotherapy Management of Cystic Fibrosis doc (2017).

Timing treatments (except emergency)

Before a feed/meal or at least 1 hour afterwards (to reduce risk of vomit/aspiration)

1. Bronchodilator nebuliser
2. Mucolytic
3. Chest physiotherapy
4. Antibiotic nebuliser

If the child is known to a specialist children's hospital, but is now in your district general hospital, contact the specialist centre for advice.

ASTHMA

Respiratory physiotherapists play an important role in identifying and managing breathing dysfunction at rest and during exercise, in children with asthma. Dysfunctional breathing symptoms often overlap and mimic asthma symptoms. The BTS/Scottish Intercollegiate Guideline Network asthma guidelines (2016) recommend breathing retraining exercises, including the Buteyko and Papworth method that use nasal and diaphragmatic breathing to establish a normal respiratory rate, volume, and pattern. A skilled physiotherapist can assess exercise-induced symptoms and identify if the limiting factor is bronchospasm, dysfunctional breathing or alternative diagnoses through observation, auscultation and spirometry. Ensure you follow the child's asthma action plan and trust policy on managing an asthma attack.

Be aware of exercise induced laryngeal obstruction, symptoms including stridor, breathlessness and upper respiratory tract (URT) discomfort during exercise, if found, refer to the appropriate specialist team.

BRONCHOSPASM

Manual chest techniques can increase bronchospasm, but sometimes benefit can outweigh risk. If the child has a lobar collapse because of secretions and bronchospasm, consider a bronchodilator nebuliser before (and possibly after) physiotherapy. Monitor for signs of increased bronchospasm: prolonged expiration, wheeze, chest tightness and dry cough, and consider adapting techniques to incorporate long expiratory vibrations and slow percussion. Avoid devices that may hyperinflate the lungs.

LONG-TERM VENTILATION

Children on long-term ventilation are assessed and treated like adults but consider:
- If the ventilator pressures or hours of use have increased, indicating greater dependence, take extra care with time off for suction and consider adding oxygen
- Ensure good mask/interface seal in noninvasive ventilation and pressure areas are intact
- Consider using ventilation during physiotherapy to reduce respiratory muscle fatigue and optimise effectiveness
- If secretions are thick, consider humidification and/or regular nebulisers. Monitor for signs of overhumidification
- For children with tracheostomies, consult the MDT for correct size of catheter and suction depth

COMPLEX NEEDS: NEUROLOGICAL CONDITIONS

Children with neurological conditions, like cerebral palsy, have increased susceptibility to respiratory infections and/or sputum retention. Respiratory physiotherapists have acute and long-term management roles to optimise respiratory function. Techniques include mucolytics, positioning, manual chest therapy, nasopharyngeal and oral suction.
   Key factors to consider:
- Establish normal respiratory baseline. Is nasal flare normal when well? Are there chronic lung changes? Are they on medication which suppresses their respiratory system and causes desaturation?

Scoliosis can alter rib biomechanics and cause hypoventilation to the underlying lung

- Children with prolonged immobility may have reduced bone density. If requiring manual chest therapy, consider on a risk versus benefit basis
- The child may be fully dependent on others for positioning, bed mobility and sitting in a chair. It is particularly important they are regularly repositioned to facilitate airway clearance, optimise V/Q matching and for postural support and development. A child may not be placed in a certain position because of past pain or poor tolerance. Retrying these positions may be important for effective treatment and to help prevent asymmetrical thoracic development, scoliosis and associated problems
- Altered tone and soft tissue laxity in the upper airway may cause obstruction characterised by stridor, tracheal tug and reduced oxygen saturations. URT secretions may also sound louder in the presence of stridor, however physiotherapy is **not** indicated. If a jaw thrust manoeuvre reduces the stridor and improves oxygen saturations, this confirms upper airway obstruction, which may require medical or surgical management
- Dysphagia and muscle weakness in the face may cause pooling of oral secretions. These do not often cause a serious medical problem but need addressing if they are causing respiratory distress or aspiration. Management includes nasopharyngeal suction, anticholinergic medication if secretions are loose and copious or mucolytics if secretions are thick. Effective secretion management is a balance between anticholinergic and mucolytics and other potential medical or surgical options. Chest physiotherapy is **not** indicated for URT secretions, but you can be a source of advice
- Weak cough or reduced cough frequency may lead to URT secretion retention. Cough-assist/manual insufflation-exsufflation (MIE) or breath stacking, using a lung volume recruitment bag, may not elicit a cough but will increase lung volumes and potentially secretion mobilisation.

NEUROMUSCULAR CONDITIONS

Neuromuscular disorders include dystrophinopathies and spinal muscular atrophy. Many children have normal intelligence but are at risk of severe respiratory infections because of muscle weakness and fatigue, which may be progressive. They are at risk of dysphagia and aspiration and may eventually require long-term ventilation. The BTS Guideline for

Respiratory Management of Children with Neuromuscular Weakness (2012) provides an overview of respiratory physiotherapy management. Signs of increased WOB may be harder to detect in these children, so pay particular attention to their respiratory rate, signs of underventilation, paradoxical abdominal movement and breathlessness. During a respiratory infection, the child's muscle strength will be reduced and take longer to recover. Physiotherapy aims are not only to treat the acute infection, but also equip the child and family to continue management at home.

It is important to assess cough strength, frequency and spontaneity. MIE, breath stacking, manual assisted cough, percussion and vibrations, respiratory adjuncts, mucolytics, humidification and positioning for $\dot{V}/\dot{Q}$ matching are all useful techniques.

Treatment considerations:

- Oxygen saturations less than 95% in air can indicate a need for airway clearance techniques
- Children with a cough peak flow (CPF) less than 270 (indicating poor cough strength) should be taught techniques to improve cough strength, for example, breath stacking and MIE. Vital capacity (as a measure of respiratory muscle strength) should be monitored regularly to assess daytime and nocturnal ventilation requirements
- MIE should be considered in weak children, unable to perform a CPF, particularly if other cough augmentation techniques are not effective
- A resuscitation bag and suction should be readily available during airway clearance techniques in hospital and at home. Sputum plugs that can be mobilised into large airways causing obstruction

ONCOLOGY

Cancer in children and young people predisposes them to viral, fungal and bacterial chest infections.

TREATMENT CONSIDERATIONS:

- Low platelet count—check for signs of active bleeding
- Mucositis (limits use of oral respiratory adjuncts because of pain)
- Peripheral neuropathies (restricts mobility)
- Lung cancer/lung metastasis—contraindicates manual chest physiotherapy and PEP/oscillatory-PEP adjuncts

SURGICAL PATIENTS

Effects of the surgery and the anaesthetic are the same as adults (see Chapter 10).

General postoperative physiotherapy includes; sitting upright, regular repositioning, mobilisation, blowing games, active cycle of breathing technique, upper limb exercises and a supported cough. Time treatments with analgesia. Optimise humidification if on oxygen therapy. Occasionally, nasopharyngeal suction is indicated, particularly with an underlying neurological/neuromuscular disorder. Ensure you follow trust protocols.

Be aware opiates depress the central nervous system.

Children, after spinal surgery, initially need to be log rolled. Some may have also had a rib excision (costectomies) —a strong caution for performing manual chest physiotherapy.

After cardiac and abdominal surgery children are at risk of developing a pleural effusion.

EXERCISE

Exercise and activity should not be underestimated. It is part of airway clearance, improves exercise tolerance, ventilation, muscle strength, function and joint movement. You have a key role, establishing an individualised exercise programme whilst in hospital, and progressing this for home.

Summary

- Respiratory assessment is the same, despite the various problems
- Establish normal baselines for long-term and complex patients
- Exercise and activity should not be underestimated
- Always communicate with the child, parents and the MDT

References

BTS/SIGN asthma guidelines, 2016. https://www.brit-thoracic.org.uk/quality-improvement/guidelines/asthma/.

BTS Guideline for Respiratory Management of Children with Neuromuscular Weakness, 2012.

Hull, J., Aniapravan, R., Chan, E., et al., 2012. British Thoracic Society guideline for respiratory management of children with neuromuscular weakness. Thorax 67, i1–i40.

NICE guidelines in Cystic Fibrosis, 2017. https://www.nice.org.uk/guidance/ng78/evidence/full-guideline-pdf-4610685853.

Pasteur, M.C., Bilton, D., Hill, A.T., on behalf of the British Thoracic Society Bronchiectasis (non-CF) Guideline Group, 2010. British Thoracic. Society guideline for non-CFbronchiectasis. Thorax 65 i1–i58.

Standards of Care and Good Clinical Practice for the Physiotherapy Management of Cystic Fibrosis doc, 2017. https://www.cysticfibrosis.org.uk/the-work-we-do/resources-for-cf-professionals/consensus-documents.

CHAPTER 17

PAEDIATRIC CRITICAL CARE

Vanessa Compton

INTRODUCTION

Paediatric critical care covers a wide age range, from premature babies to 16 years and over, with a multitude of conditions. With such a varied caseload, you must understand the changes in anatomic and physiological functioning from prematurity to adulthood (see Chapter 3). Detailed respiratory assessment applies to all, regardless of age and condition. Targeted assessment skills can be used, depending on condition and presentation, to identify problems and devise appropriate treatment plans. Treatments should not be routine but planned after careful consideration and clinical reasoning.

AIMS

By the end of this chapter you should be able to:

- Describe paediatric specific issues in critical care
- Discuss goals of treatment in paediatric critical care

THE ENVIRONMENT

Paediatric critical care describes the environment where enhanced observation, monitoring or interventions can take place.

There are three levels of care (Paediatric Intensive Care Standards)

Level 1—Basic critical care (standard high-dependency unit [HDU] at ward level)

Level 2—Intermediate critical care (HDU or paediatric intensive care unit [PICU])

Level 3—Advanced critical care with subgroups: advanced 1 to 5 (PICU)

Critical care units are full of technology, equipment, people and loud noises and are frightening for children and parents. Parents have 24-hour access, and are likely be at the bedside, if their child is unwell. Careful explanations before interventions, including likely outcomes and possible adverse reactions, are essential. Parents may wish to stay during interventions, talk to them, reassure them and the child, and try to be calm and confident. Use the knowledge of the highly skilled medical and nursing staff by asking questions.

THE POPULATION

Assessment

Conduct a thorough assessment, children are at high risk of deterioration, have complex needs, so vigilance is essential.

In addition to usual assessment (see Paediatric wards, Chapter 16), there are considerations specific to the child's condition and presentation.

Assessment Specific to Critical Care

Subjective Assessment

Ask nursing staff/parents for history that may affect the patient's overall condition, including gestational age, previous episodes of ventilation, home O_2, normal pattern of breathing and home physiotherapy regimes. Thus a clear baseline is established, that is, what is normal for the child?

Why is the patient on critical care?

Have they been stable since admission?

Bedside nursing staff will be able to tell you about the current condition, behaviour and plans. Trends and patterns should be noted.

Objective Assessment

Cardiovascular system
- Patients may have labile blood pressure, abnormal heart rhythms, alterations in heart rate, poor perfusion or temperature change.
- It is important to know how much cardiovascular (inotropic) support a patient is receiving and if it is escalating or weaning.

Perfusion
- Capillary refill time should be less than 2 seconds; this is performed over the manubriosternum, not peripherally

Ventilation

- Does the patient have an artificial airway? (endotracheal tube/tracheostomy). Note the type, size, length and position of the artificial airway to ensure correct suction depth and security of tube
- Assess the level of ventilation and fraction of inspired oxygen the child requires. Look carefully at trends over the previous 24 hours. Is the child weaning, static or are their ventilation/oxygen requirements escalating?
- If ventilated on pressure-controlled ventilation note the tidal volume. A decrease in tidal volume can indicate atelectasis, consolidation, pleural effusion or pneumothorax. Persistent decrease in tidal volume will result in compromised gas exchange. It can be used as an objective marker to assess the efficacy of treatment.

Blood Gases (see Appendix 2)

Chest x-ray

- Use to support your assessment findings but remember children change very quickly.

Central nervous system

- Are they sedated and/or receiving muscle relaxants?
- What is their level of consciousness?
- How do they respond to handling? (So you can plan and assess your treatment.)
- Are they in pain? If ventilated they may need extrasedation/muscle relaxant before treatment to lessen adverse reactions.
- Are they moving? Is this movement appropriate? Are lines/attachments at risk?

Fluid balance

- Do they have a significant positive or negative fluid balance? This can affect secretion viscosity and make ventilation and secretion clearance difficult. Look for signs and symptoms that the child is dehydrated or fluid overloaded.
- Saline or hypertonic saline nebulisers can be given before treatment if secretions are tenacious. If they are spontaneously breathing, and not nil by mouth, encourage them to drink.

Risk assessment

- Identify and record all lines, drains and equipment to prevent any being dislodged while handling.
- Identify risks to treatment, such as cardiovascular system (CVS) instability and plan your actions.
- Moving critically ill patients is necessary, make sure there are enough staff and the correct equipment available.

Clinical Reasoning

Clinical reasoning in critical care is complex with often incomplete and rapidly changing data. Understand the risks related to the specific disease and medical treatment and make sure that the risk and benefit to the patient is determined.

Clinical intervention and considerations

Goals for physiotherapy in critical care

- Decrease secretion retention
- Maintain or recruit lung volume to reduce atelectasis
- Improve lung compliance
- Improve gas exchange
- Reduce airway resistance and work of breathing
- Improve respiratory muscle strength
- Improve/maintain joint range, muscle strength and mobility
- Reduce patient morbidity, length of critical care and hospital stay

Paediatric critical care considerations

See Chapter 9 Treatments.

TREATMENTS FOR SPUTUM RETENTION, ATELECTASIS	
TREATMENT	CONSIDERATIONS
Percussion and vibrations	<ul><li>Platelet count</li><li>Fractures</li><li>Bone density</li><li>Bronchospasm</li><li>Cardiovascular system (CVS) instability</li></ul>
Manual hyperinflation	<ul><li>Note patient's ventilator pressures and O_2 requirement before commencing treatment</li><li>CVS instability, increased intrathoracic pressure produces decreased venous return</li><li>Pneumothorax</li></ul>

TREATMENTS FOR SPUTUM RETENTION, ATELECTASIS—cont'd

TREATMENT	CONSIDERATIONS
Positioning	• Consider anatomical differences in children (see Chapter 3) • Head down tip will increase diaphragmatic load, increase intrathoracic pressure and increase risk of reflux/ aspiration—use if necessary, but with care • Lines and attachments
Mobilisation	• Sedation effects • Pain • Psychological effect for patients and carers • Potential increase in oxygen consumption • CVS instability
Incentive spirometry	• Requires child's cooperation • Pain in the child's mouth because of mucositis
Assisted coughing/manual insufflation/exsufflation	• Requires child's cooperation • Discomfort • Desaturation • Pneumothorax
Positive pressure devices	• Requires child's cooperation • Discomfort • Desaturation • Pneumothorax
Deep breathing exercises	• Requires child's cooperation • Use games/play
Suction	• Correct depth? • Timing (feeds/meds that may decrease level of consciousness
NaCl installation	• Never use routinely • Avoid with premature neonates • May be warmed if child has reactive airways • Follow trust guidelines
Bronchoalveolar lavage (BAL)	• Therapeutic BAL • Diagnostic BAL • Follow trust guidelines
Nebulisers	• Hypertonic NaCl may cause bronchospasm • Salbutamol will increase heart rate

Continued

TREATMENTS FOR SPUTUM RETENTION, ATELECTASIS—cont'd

TREATMENT	CONSIDERATIONS
Mucolytics, e.g., dornase alpha/ acetylcysteine	• May cause inflammation of the mouth, chest tightness and pulmonary haemorrhage
Hyoscine/ glycopyrrolate	Normal dose may need altering or stopping if secretion viscosity increases

TREATMENTS THAT MAINTAIN OR IMPROVE LUNG VOLUME, VENTILATION AND LUNG COMPLIANCE

TREATMENT	CONSIDERATIONS
Manual chest clearance techniques	• Often more beneficial when used with MHI and positioning
Manual hyperinflation (MHI)	• Use correct size bag to prevent overinflation/ pneumothorax • Take care if cardiovascular system (CVS) instability • Monitor observations throughout • Can be used for lung recruitment and to improve compliance
Positioning	• Aids recruitment of specific areas of the lungs
Closed suction	• Prevents loss of positive end expiratory pressure during suction • Maintains oxygen delivery • Assess response to closed suction without disconnection. If closed suction is not enough, consider MHI with closed suction. If so, two people should perform these treatments • Monitor observations throughout
High frequency oscillatory ventilation (HFOV)	• Care needed when disconnecting from ventilator to perform MHI, suction or to change patient position • Endotracheal tubes may be clamped to reduce loss of surface area recruitment • Pre- and postoxygenate • Recruitment manoeuvres may need to be after physiotherapy – refer to your trust policy

TREATMENTS THAT MAINTAIN OR IMPROVE LUNG VOLUME, VENTILATION AND LUNG COMPLIANCE—cont'd

TREATMENT	CONSIDERATIONS
Breath stacking, breath augmentation, cough assist or intermittent positive pressure breathing	• Used for lung recruitment • Poor synchrony because of pain and discomfort • Monitor observations throughout • Pneumothorax

Volume loss can occur as a result of atelectasis and lung collapse because of airway obstruction or by compression of the lung because of pneumothorax or pleural fluid. You must ascertain the cause to decide if physiotherapy is appropriate.

TREATMENTS THAT IMPROVE VENTILATION AND PERFUSION

TREATMENT	CONSIDERATIONS
Positioning	• Infants will have reflux, if endotracheal tube is uncuffed, there is a risk of aspiration • Do not routinely use head down gravity assisted positions? • Prone positioning decreases work of breathing and improves ventiliation/perfusion matching • Prone position can be used with any size child providing they are fully monitored • Ensure manual handling guidelines are followed

TREATMENTS TO REDUCE AIRWAY RESISTANCE AND WORK OF BREATHING

TREATMENT	CONSIDERATIONS
Manual hyperinflation, positioning, suction, manual techniques, saline	• Highly effective if secretions are sole cause • Can exacerbate reactive airways and lead to increased bronchospasm • Ensure medication is available should this occur • Warm NaCl if bronchospasm present • Do not treat if suspected inhaled foreign body
Nebulisers	• In acute exacerbations of asthma, nebulisers alone may not be enough and intravenous medications may be required • Salbutamol increases heart rate

Continued

TREATMENTS TO REDUCE AIRWAY RESISTANCE AND WORK OF BREATHING—cont'd

TREATMENT	CONSIDERATIONS
Manual decompressions (prolonged expiratory pressure on the child's chest)	• Used for air trapping • Close monitoring of cardiovascular system throughout
HELIOX—An inert gas containing helium and 21% (or 35%) oxygen Administered via nonrebreather mask or endotracheal or tracheostomy tube	• Reduces turbulent flow in airways and reduces work of breathing • Used with conditions, such as asthma, bronchiectasis, bronchiolitis, croup, cystic fibrosis, epiglottitis and postextubation stridor • Used in conjunction with chest physiotherapy techniques to ensure therapy is maximised • No known side effects

It is important to decide whether increased airway resistance is caused by retained secretions, bronchospasm, airway obstruction or inflammation or a combination of these.

TREATMENTS TO OPTIMISE OXYGENATION AND VENTILATION

TREATMENT	CONSIDERATIONS
Effective oxygen delivery	• Titrate to maintain pulse oximetry (SpO_2) levels to prescribed levels • Oxygenation may need to be increased during or after physiotherapy, particularly if gravity assisted positioning for drainage is used because head downs positions will splint the diaphragm and increase work of breathing • Consider humidification
Positioning	• Communication with nursing staff and parents is essential to ensure implementation

TREATMENTS TO IMPROVE RESPIRATORY MUSCLE STRENGTH

TREATMENT	CONSIDERATIONS
Ventilator weaning plans/ strategies	• Must be very patient specific and involve the multidisciplinary team
Positive expiratory pressure, inspiratory and expiratory muscle trainers	• Muscles require overloading (tiring) to obtain a training response, so note when your patients may tire quickly • Care with asthmatic patients

TREATMENTS TO IMPROVE/MAINTAIN JOINT RANGE, MUSCLE STRENGTH AND MOBILITY

TREATMENT	CONSIDERATIONS
Splinting	• Maintains joint range in children heavily sedated for long periods • Monitor pressure areas
Passive movements	• Parents can be taught passive movements and gentle massage to encourage family centred care • Take care with lines and attachments • Consider bone density to prevent fractures (in complex needs children who do not weight bear and have low bone density) • Be respectful of privacy and dignity, while performing passive movements
Active or active assisted movements	• Help maintain muscle strength and mobility, boosts morale – incorporate with play • If it is safe, teach parents/carers
Early mobilisation	• Assists recovery and psychological well-being • Consider while still ventilated after full risk assessment • Ensure adequate staff to mobilise safely

It is important to maintain joint range and mobility when in critical care. Patients can have a long stay becoming debilitated. Critical illness neuropathy can be a common side effect if ventilated for more than 7 days.

TREATMENTS TO REDUCE MORBIDITY OF A CRITICAL CARE ADMISSION

TREATMENT	CONSIDERATIONS
Mobilisation	• Early assessment, treatment and mobilisation essential • Caution with lines, drains and attachments • Adequate pain relief
Infection control	• Follow trust protocols for infection control, hand hygiene etc

GENERAL CONSIDERATIONS/CONTRAINDICATIONS TO TREATMENT

- Undrained pneumothorax
- CVS instability
- Head injury
- Recent pulmonary surgery
- Bullae
- Bronchospasm
- Presence of subcutaneous emphysema
- Coagulopathy
- Conditions that are secondary to inflammation may not respond to physiotherapy interventions for example, bronchiolitis/influenza/acute pneumonia/consolidation.

SPECIAL CONSIDERATIONS IN CRITICAL CARE

NonInvasive Ventilation (NIV)
See Chapter 8 Respiratory failure

Considerations
- Correct fitting of interfaces is essential to avoid asynchrony because of leaks and poor triggering. It will also improve compliance and prevent skin breakdown
- The patient may not tolerate being removed from noninvasive ventilation (NIV) for physiotherapy or pressure relief. Bag-valve-mask

ventilation may be needed. Ensure a competent member of nursing staff is present to assist with treatments
- Pressure relief is required at regular intervals (see individual unit policies), usually 3 to 4 hourly.
- Pressure relief must be complete removal of the mask and head gear. Skin should be checked for marking under the mask and head straps. Alternative masks may be used for pressure relief if necessary. Pressure relieving tape or barrier creams should be used to prevent pressure areas
- Use NIV with caution if a patient presents with nausea/vomiting, excessive secretions or a decrease in conscious level

Cardiac surgery
Considerations
- Be aware that patients may have an alteration of blood flow to the lungs (too much or too little)
- Make a note of acceptable pulse oximetry (SpO_2) for patient if palliative surgery is performed or a partial repair. Manual hyperinflation (MHI) with oxygen/air mixer may be required if the patient has a duct dependant cardiac lesion requiring Prostin (refer to your trust policy)
- Be aware of possible cardiac shunting; this may redirect blood flow preferentially to the lungs, or the heart, causing swinging O_2 saturations
- Patients may return from theatre with an open sternum; modified positioning will be necessary and manual techniques should only be used after discussion with a senior clinician
- Patients are often highly unstable; justify any intervention and monitor closely throughout always seek help from an experienced clinician if in any doubt
- Patient may require bolus of muscle relaxant and sedation before treatment if unstable

Premature Infants
Babies born under 36-weeks' gestation are defined as premature. Treatments should only be undertaken after careful assessment and you are competent to do so.

Considerations
- Often require minimal handling (usually 6–8 hours between nursing care)

- Poor temperature control, so do not leave the incubators open for long periods
- May be under ultraviolet lights for jaundice, which can be turned off during physiotherapy
- Handle careful they have delicate skin and no subcutaneous fat
- Endotracheal tubes are small and can easily block/dislodge
- Do not use saline as routine as airway blockage and removal of surfactant can occur. If absolutely necessary, use in small amounts (0.1–0.2 mL)
- Support the head during manual techniques
- Accept lower SpO2 because of foetal circulation and lung prematurity (check target range; usually >88%)
- Accept altered parameters for arterial blood gases (pH >7.25 is acceptable)
- Surfactant therapy may be given; do not suction, unless absolutely necessary, for at least 6 hours after it has been administered

Bronchoalveolar Lavage

Bronchoalveolar lavage (BAL) may be to clear airways, most commonly to remove mucous plugging, but also smoke inhalation and removal of sooty plaques. BALs are also used for diagnostic sputum samples. Trust policy should be followed when performing a BAL, either as a treatment technique or for diagnostic sample.

Considerations

- Careful consideration is required for patients with reactive airways (e.g., asthma). You may need to administer bronchodilators before and/or after the procedure (refer to your trust policy)
- May cause bleeding in patients with low platelets/coagulopathies

Head Injury

Traumatic brain injuries (TBIs) are common in children and remain one of the largest causes of mortality and disability. Initial management of TBI patients focuses on the prevention of secondary brain injury; close monitoring, treatment of hypoxia, intracranial hypertension, ensuring systemic resuscitation and multisystem stabilisation. Working with the multidisciplinary team (MDT) when planning and performing physiotherapy to prevent possible hypoxia and hypertension.

Considerations
- Position supine with head elevation of 30 degrees
- Log roll and neck immobilisation, until spinal cord injury excluded
- Nasopharyngeal suction contraindicated if evidence of basal skull fracture
- Cluster care to minimise handling
- Preoxygenate the patient
- Instil lignocaine into endotracheal tube before suction to prevent cough and subsequent intracranial pressure (ICP) spike
- Bolus sedation and muscle relaxant if ICP unstable
- Gentle hyperinflation can be used to reduce ICP if required. Always use an end tidal CO_2 monitor in bagging circuit
- Use closed suction if positive end expiratory pressure greater than 6 cm H2O
- Always use the correct suction depth
- Monitor ICP/cerebral perfusion pressure throughout and record any changes
- Constantly reassess during and after each intervention

Inhaled nitric oxide

Inhaled nitric oxide (iNO) is commonly used in specialist units as a specific pulmonary vasodilator to treat pulmonary hypertension and hypoxic respiratory failure.

Considerations
- During MHI, iNO must be added to the circuit
- Risk for pregnant workers will be addressed in Trust policies

Extra Corporeal Membrane Oxygenation

Extra corporeal membrane oxygenation (ECMO) is an artificial lung that diffuses oxygen into the blood and continuously pumps this blood into and around the body. It is delivered at designated ECMO centres and supports patients (who have the potential to recover) with life-threatening respiratory and cardiovascular compromise. ECMO supports the patient through the disease process, whilst therapies to take place to aid recovery.

There are two types of ECMO:
- Veno-arterial ECMO—bypasses the lungs by delivering oxygen directly to the blood. This supports the heart by delivering this blood, under pressure, into the arterial system to provide a mean blood

pressure. This has the effect of resting the heart and lungs allowing recovery to take place.

- Veno-venous ECMO—supports the lungs by delivery of oxygenated blood into the body bypassing the lungs. There is no support for blood pressure in this mode.

All physiotherapeutic treatments can be used but may require adaptation. Treatments often include MHI, manual techniques, suction, positioning, lavage, optimising lung volumes, splinting, passive movement and active rehabilitation.

Communication between the physiotherapist, bedside nurse and ECMO specialist is essential for safe and effective treatments.

Considerations

Document ECMO type and position of ECMO cannulae. Awareness of both external and internal position of the cannulae is necessary, as well as their security.

- If the chest is open, modify positioning and use posterior vibrations if necessary
- Is the ECMO flow stable? What is affecting it?
- Monitor and assess coagulation and bleeding. Bear in mind the circuit is heparinised
- Be aware that positioning, MHI, vibrations and coughing may lead to a drop in ECMO flow. Treatments can be modified. Proceed with caution at all times

---

Paediatric Critical Care Key Messages

- Be thorough and methodical
- Gather appropriate information
- Consider preexisting and new pathologies
- Work closely with the experienced nursing and medical staff. If in doubt—ask for help
- These patients are more prone to atelectasis/retained secretions. They fatigue and deteriorate quickly—you must respond promptly
- Frequently reassess your patient
- Always communicate with the patient, parents and the multidisciplinary team

CHAPTER 18

WORKING IN THE COMMUNITY WITH THE ACUTELY ILL RESPIRATORY PATIENT

Helen Ashcroft-Kelso

INTRODUCTION

Community physiotherapists work with a wide range of patient conditions outside of the usual hospital setting with minimal resources. They are essential in providing care to those for whom access to hospital services is challenging, perhaps because of the effort or inconvenience of travel. They have a unique opportunity to tailor the treatment they prescribe to the patient's home environment, resources and home care team. This chapter considers the management of the acutely ill respiratory patients in the community setting.

If you are unsure about the patient's stability or safety, while treating them at home, call for appropriate help, even that of the emergency services if necessary. See Fig. 18.1 for more information. If an emergency requires paramedic and ambulance support, you must be clear, what the parameters for escalation of care are, including any prearranged ceilings of care.

AIMS

By the end of the chapter you should:
- Understand the complexities of the community environment
- Understand how to adapt an assessment for the community patient
- Identify signs of deterioration
- Understand how to treat the acutely unwell community patient
- Know when to refer to specialist services
- Know when to escalate to urgent care

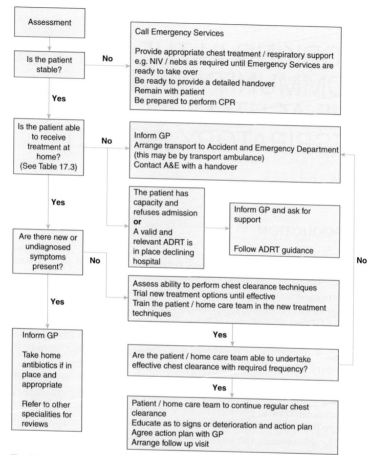

Fig. 18.1 • **Decision making flowchart for the community patient.** *ADRT,* Advanced decision to refuse treatment; *CPR,* Cardiopulmonary resuscitation; *GP,* general practitioner; *NIV,* noninvasive ventilation.

THE ENVIRONMENT

Sometimes, it is more appropriate to assess the patient in the environment in which they live. Community treatment provides privacy and conserves energy for patients who are very unwell. With some limitations in access to medical equipment, treatment options can be reduced, and creativity is required to produce success. If a home care team is in place, and they are able to undertake a given treatment safely and effectively, thus can contribute to the treatment choice. Specific training and education, relevant to the environment, will be needed. Working within a patient's home requires sensitivity from you, if and when, you are invited into a very personal setting. You may encounter family and carer dynamics, in a way, not apparent in other healthcare settings.

THE POPULATION

Patients requiring community physiotherapy are varied but can include the very unwell and severely disabled. Some maybe at the end of their lives and you can offer them more dignity in the privacy of their own home during treatment.

For example:

The very breathless patient, perhaps with chronic obstructive pulmonary disease (COPD), may find travelling to appointments simply too tiring.

Patients with bronchiectasis, requiring support with chest clearance, may benefit from preserving their energy to participate maximally in their treatment.

Patients with both physical and learning disabilities may find the unfamiliar hospital environment distressing.

Neuromuscular conditions, such as motor neurone disease (MND) or multiple sclerosis, may simply be too frail.

These conditions place patients at high risk of chest infection and respiratory failure is often the cause of death. Recognising both chronic and acute respiratory deterioration and optimising care can prevent avoidable hospital admissions, positively impact on quality of life and improve survival.

PREPARING FOR THE VISIT

Establishing a number of things in advance of the visit helps you decide what medical equipment to take and improves safety for both you and the patient. Table 18.1 gives examples of things that you should consider

CONSIDERATION	RELEVANCE
Prescribed target oxygen saturation range	Usually ≥94% In some cases, like chronic respiratory failure, COPD and severe disease this could be 88%–92%
Home oxygen therapy Long-term oxygen therapy (LTOT)	What is the prescribed flow rate of oxygen? • While sleeping • Awake at rest • On ambulation Is there flexibility to increase this during periods of acute ill health? Note: NMD patients should not be offered LTOT, unless there is comorbidity.
Home respiratory management	Do they have: • Antibiotics at home for emergency use • Nebulisers • Respiratory support, such as CPAP or NIV • Tracheostomy • Chest clearance devices
Palliative care	Does the patient have: • Symptom management via syringe drivers Advanced decision to refuse treatment (ADRT): Refer to the ADRT information later • 'Just in case' kit of anticipatory medications
Family members and care teams	How many staff make up the care package? How many family members could you expect to encounter? Who is next of kin? Does anyone have a current power of attorney for health and welfare?
Personal safety working alone	Are the area/family/carers well known to you? Are there any existing safeguarding concerns? Are there any pets, such as dogs in the home? How will you get help if you need it? – Buddy system?

TABLE 18.1 THINGS TO KNOW BEFORE YOU GO

COPD, Chronic obstructive pulmonary disease; CPAP, continuous pressure airway breathing; NIV, MND, motor neurone disease; noninvasive ventilation.

ASSESSMENT

Much of the assessment described in Chapter 2 remains appropriate in the community environment. The National Early Warning Score (NEWS)2 tool is not yet validated for community use but can be used alongside your assessment to monitor changes in an acutely unwell patient, determine the seriousness of their condition and when communicating with other healthcare professionals (RCP, 2017). Advice for the community environment, particularly the neuromuscular patient follows (Tables 18.2–18.4).

B—Breathing

In the home, you may find that the patient is most comfortable sitting on a sofa, however in this sitting position, you may not be able to auscultate the lung bases or observe the chest wall movement. Consider repositioning them with additional pillows or asking them to move to another seat, during which time you can also assess their mobility level.

Assume that we have repositioned patient M

Pulse oximetry

Having pulse oximetry (SpO$_2$) is really useful when assessing a community patient, but you must know the patient's target oxygen saturation range. This can be a deciding factor in whether or not to call for emergency assistance if they are acutely unwell.

C—Circulation

Heart rate may be raised because of respiratory distress and settle when the underlying cause for example, retained secretions is resolved. Cold and clammy hands may be identified during a handshake and capillary refill, a measure needing no equipment, may give an indication of their fluid level (Chapter 2 Assessment).

Back to Patient M:

For patient M, a deeper breath reveals that there are some crackles in the upper respiratory tract. A respiratory rate of 20 does not score on the NEWS2 assessment, however, clinical judgement tells you that this is perhaps more rapid than usual for a patient without underlying lung disease. SpO2 of 94% scores a 1, and heart rate of 95 increases the score to 2. You have already noticed that the patient is agitated by secretions and cough, which may be contributing the slight increase in heart rate and respiratory rate.

Using Fig. 18.1—currently patient M is well enough to remain at home and it is reasonable to continue with your assessment and provide some treatment, before reassessing the NEWS2 score. Clearing secretions effectively may normalise the score in this case.

D—Disability
Mobilisation

You should assess the patient's mobility and enable them to mobilise as much as they can in their home. Use appropriate aids for mobility to maintain their general health and well-being, it will also benefit chest clearance.

E—Environment

In addition to 'Exposure', consider 'Environment'. Assessment of the home environment includes the available equipment, space and support team ability to provide the required treatment. Is the carer physically able, or are they frail themselves? The confidence and ability of the care team can, at times, determine the treatment choice.

COMMUNITY INTERVENTIONS AND REFERRALS

Advanced Care Planning

Patients with existing respiratory compromise are at high risk of serious deterioration during a chest infection. The National Institute for Care and Health Excellence (NICE) guidance recommends that antibiotics are prescribed immediately if a chest infection is suspected. Delay in assessment can delay antibiotic prescribing, so consider talking to the general practitioner (GP) about prescribing a rescue pack of antibiotics to be kept at home. The patient should be educated to recognise their signs of a chest infection; a change in colour, volume or purulence of secretions compared to their normal, or perhaps breathlessness and fatigue, as a signal to take this medication appropriately. They must understand that if they begin to use the medication, they must contact their GP immediately for assessment, and management of the side effects from taking antibiotics.

Onward Referral

Treating a community patient regularly may mean that you are the first to become aware of changes in their condition. Remember, you can consult a range of specialist health professionals for advice and potentially refer the patient to. If you are unsure always, talk to your supervisor.

Advanced decisions to refuse treatment

Advance decisions to refuse treatment (ADRTs) (N.H.S. England 2013) are documented in writing, signed by the patient and this signature is witnessed. People who are aged over 18 years, and have capacity, are entitled to make decisions about their care. Once in place, all health-care professions are required to follow the ADRT. If you are aware that a patient has an ADRT you must see it, to be sure that it exists, and check that it is valid and applicable as soon as possible. ADRTs should give very clear statements regarding the care that the patient does not want in specific circumstances. For example, in the event of a cardiac arrest, the patient does not wish to receive cardiopulmonary resuscitation. Discuss ADRTs with your supervisor before you visit the patient to plan how you will manage the situation in which the ADRT must be implemented.

TABLE 18.2 COMMUNITY INTERVENTIONS AND REFERRALS

PRESENTING COMPLAINT	ADVICE AND TREATMENT OPTIONS	COMMENTS
Airway		
Bulbar weakness	Assess peak cough flow regularly, as it impacts on secretion retention Consider oral suction Consider referral to specialist AHPs for assessment and advice: • Dietician • Speech and language therapist • Respiratory specialist physiotherapist	Identification at an early stage can help prevent potential aspiration and chest infection. **Caution**: Excessive suction can cause dryness of the mouth
Drooling	Saliva volume can be managed with medications. Consider referral to: • GP • Palliative care team • Specialist nurse	Prophylaxis is key. Preventing aspiration is preferable to treating its effects
	Consider oral suction	**Caution**: Excessive suction can cause dryness of the mouth

Continued

TABLE 18.2	COMMUNITY INTERVENTIONS AND REFERRALS—cont'd	
PRESENTING COMPLAINT	ADVICE AND TREATMENT OPTIONS	COMMENTS
Breathing		
Secretion retention	Assess the technique of the patient/home care team in the current treatment method. Is it effective? Trial alternative treatment techniques and reassess Consider referral to the specialist respiratory centre for assessment if treatments remain ineffective	If the patient requires a new treatment method, and has a home care team supporting them, the home care team must be provided with education and training to enable them to treat the patient effectively and report any difficulties Note: Patients on NIV may need to use it between cycles of chest clearance for relief of breathlessness
Breathing difficulty	Always call for help if severe Use furniture, equipment and cushions in the patient's home to teach: • Positions of ease • Pacing • Energy conservation Has the patient taken/could they take prescribed medications e.g., inhalers	Consider pharmacist referral if patients cannot take their medications safely
	Neuromuscular patients: do not lay the patient flat. Support them into an upright position Ensure the head is supported to maintain the airway	Patients with respiratory muscle weakness become more breathless in lying Patients with neck weakness may require a head and neck support to maintain a patent airway
	If the airway is patent and NIV is already available, apply the NIV	NIV will provide breathing support required to relieve the work of breathing

TABLE 18.2	COMMUNITY INTERVENTIONS AND REFERRALS— cont'd	
PRESENTING COMPLAINT	ADVICE AND TREATMENT OPTIONS	COMMENTS
Increased dependence on NIV	Refer to the specialist respiratory centre if there is a change in the patients use of NIV, e.g., time/length of use, mask fit. They may consider providing a backup ventilator/ appropriate masks, methods of mask pressure relief	Palliative medications for relief of breathlessness may enable breaks from NIV Pressure areas are of grave concern because they eventually prevent NIV use and increase mortality risk
Panic	Treat the underlying cause Call for help as appropriate	Breathlessness management and pacing work well with some patients (e.g., COPD) Patients with MND may have a 'Just in Case' kit. The carer will be trained to use the 'emergency medications for carers' which can treat: • Panic • Choking • Breathlessness The kit also includes a section of emergency medications for use by appropriately trained healthcare professionals
Disability		
Immobility	Assess and provide equipment to enable mobility and ensure the patient can: • Wash • Dress • Use the toileting • Eat and drink May require an increased package of care, referral to social work or occupational therapy	Local teams may provide rapid equipment delivery. Some bridge care until a care package can be established, reducing hospital admissions

AHPs, Allied Health Professionals; *COPD,* chronic obstructive pulmonary disease; *MND,* motor neurone disease; *NIV,* noninvasive ventilation.

TABLE 18.3 FACTORS TO CONSIDER REGARDING SAFEST PLACE FOR CARE IN ACUTE ILLNESS

FACTOR	TREAT AT HOME	TREAT IN HOSPITAL
General condition	Normal level	Sudden and significant deterioration
Significant comorbidity (particularly respiratory and cardiac diseases)	No	Yes
Previous hospitalisations	May be more likely to need or want hospital-based care	
Social circumstances	Good	Living alone/not coping and aids cannot be provided to correct immediately
Respiratory rate	≤20	>20
Pulse oximetry (SpO_2)	Within target SpO_2 range	Below target SpO_2 range
Acute confusion	No	Yes
Worsening peripheral oedema	No	Yes
Level of consciousness	Normal	Impaired—more drowsy or difficult to rouse

(Modified from: NICE, 2018. Chronic obstructive pulmonary disease in over 16s: diagnosis and management. Available from: https://www.nice.org.uk/guidance/ng115/chapter/Recommendations [Accessed Feb 2019])

TABLE 18.4	ADDITIONAL CONSIDERATIONS FOR NEUROMUSCULAR/VENTILATED PATIENTS	
BASELINE DIAGNOSIS	MND PATIENTS ARE MORE LIKELY TO REQUIRE HOSPITAL ADMISSION	
Bulbar symptoms	Absent or mild impairment	Moderate or severe impairment
NIV pattern of use (if already in use)	Using regularly with no significant usage pattern change	Not using/significant change in usage pattern
Home care team provide adequate treatment frequency and effect	Able	Unable
Advanced decision to refuse treatment (ADRT)	In place—does not wish to be admitted to hospital	Not in place/in place and desires hospital admission

MND, Motor neurone disease; *NIV*, noninvasive ventilation.

Summary

- Patients are increasingly being cared for in the community setting
- Remember, the assessment and treatment skills that you already have remain useful and relevant in the patient's home
- Thorough preparation will ensure visits go smoothly
- Community care can significantly improve patient quality of life, family experience and reduce pressures on other healthcare services

References

NICE, 2008. Self-limiting Respiratory Tract and Ear Infections– Antibiotic Prescribing Overview. http://pathways.nice.org.uk/pathways/self-limiting-respiratory-tract-and-ear-infections-antibiotic-prescribing. Accessed Feb 2019.

N.H.S. England, 2013. Advanced Decision to Refuse Treatment: a Guide for Healthcare Professionals. Available from: https://www.england.nhs.uk/improvement-hub/publication/advance-decisions-to-refuse-treatment-a-guide-for-health-and-social-care-professionals/. [Accessed 29th April 2019]

NICE, 2018. Chronic Obstructive Pulmonary Disease in over 16s: Diagnosis and Management. Available from https://www.nice.org.uk/guidance/ng115/chapter/Recommendations. [Accessed Feb 2019].

Royal College of Physicians (RCP), 2017. National Early Warning Score (NEWS) 2: Standardising the Assessment of Acute-Illness Severity in the NHS. RCP, London. Updated report of a working party.

CHAPTER 19

CASE STUDIES

This chapter contains a number of case studies written by authors and editors. Work through those suitable for your learning needs.

Do not worry if the information given or presentation differs – this is all part of the learning process.

CASE STUDY 1: ADULT INTENSIVE CARE

History
A 34-year-old man admitted 4 days ago for nasogastric feeding. Transferred to intensive care unit (ICU) 3 days ago, following respiratory arrest.

Past medical history
A 15-year history of anorexia and depression; previous admissions for nutritional management.

Drug History
Citalopram.

Observation/examination
The patient is supine in bed. The nursing staff report the patient only arrived on the unit an hour ago and they have not suctioned him yet. The patient is cachexic; his weight has been estimated at 35 kg.

A: Intubated and ventilated via endotracheal tube

B: Pressure Support (PS) 25, PEEP 10 cmH$_2$O, RR 30, TV 300 mL, PAP 36,

FiO$_2$ 0.6, SpO$_2$ 92%,

ABGs: pH 7.36, PaO$_2$ 7.39, PaCO$_2$ 4.92, HCO$_3^-$ 22.0, BE –1.0

Ausc.: Decreased breath sounds throughout right lung

Palpation: Expansion, left >right

C: HR 100, BP 100/70 mmHg, Temp. 38° C

Renal: UO 40 mL, Fluid balance +900 mL

D: AVCPU

Propofol, fentanyl

E: Arterial line, peripheral access, urinary catheter

You have been asked to see this patient urgently as he was found to have a right-sided 'white out' on the postintubation chest x-ray (CXR).

Questions

1. What is the patient's main problem?
2. What will be your treatment plan?
3. What considerations might you need to consider before treatment?
4. How will you know if your treatment is effective?

Answers

1. Aspiration to the right lung. The patient's NG tube has migrated from his stomach allowing the aspiration of NG feed.
2. Treatment plan:
   a. Reposition the patient in left side-lying to aid drainage of secretions.
   b. Suction to clear secretions.
   c. Manual hyperinflation (MHI) to reinflate right lung.
3. Considerations:

   PEEP: PEEP of ≥10 cmH$_2$O

   High PAP: This patient is requiring high levels of PS and PEEP to maintain adequate gaseous exchange.

   Low body mass index (BMI): Normally a patient will be ventilated to achieve a tidal volume of 6 to 8 mL per kg. Care needs to be taken with positioning to avoid pressure area problems.

   Low BP: This BP may be acceptable for this patient because of his low BMI.
4. Ask for a repeat CXR and ABGs following treatment.

CASE STUDY 2: PAEDIATRIC INTENSIVE CARE

You are called to a 9-year-old girl on paediatric intensive care unit with asthma, admitted with respiratory distress.

Telephone History

- Upper respiratory tract infection for 2 days, increasing inhaler use
- Intubated, ventilated, sedated and paralysed, size 4.5 nasal endotracheal (ET) tube
- On intravenous (IV) salbutamol, steroids and antibiotics
- Ventilation—pressure control 24/3; 18 breaths per minute; FiO_2 0.6
- ABGs—pH 7.2, PaO_2 10 kPa, $PaCO_2$ 9.3 kPa, BE +3
- Vital signs—HR 120 beats per minute, BP 140/70 mmHg, SpO_2 92%, temperature 38.3° C
- Auscultation—mild wheeze, decreased air entry right lower zone, crackles throughout
- Patient supine, head slightly elevated
- Suction—thick mucopurulent secretions
- CXR—2 hours ago, showing right lower lobe collapse, hyperinflated left lung and gas in stomach.

Questions

1. Is this an appropriate call out?
2. Analyse the ABG
3. What could your treatment be?
4. What other treatments might you consider?
5. What else could you consider with the nursing staff?

Answers

1. Yes—retained secretions and CXR changes, monitor wheeze.
2. ABG:
   Borderline hypoxic
   Partially compensated respiratory acidosis.
3. Potential treatments:
   Left side-lying, flat or head up
   MHI—low PEEP (minimise air trapping)
   Slow percussion and vibrations (monitor wheeze)
   Saline
   Suction (+/-vibrations)
   Titrate FiO_2 to keep SpO_2 above 93%.
4. Other treatment options:
   Bronchoalveolar lavage for acute lobar collapse—if wheeze allows
   Right side-lying and MHI with vibrations/holds to decrease hyperinflation in left lung (manual decompressions).

5. Consider:
   NG tube on free drainage allows gas to escape from stomach—will
      aid diaphragm excursion
   Optimise humidification and fluids.

CASE STUDY 3: MEDICAL WARD

History
A 58-year-old woman with chronic obstructive pulmonary disease
(COPD), admitted via Accident and Emergency complaining of 1-week
history of short of breath (SOB), cough productive of purulent sputum,
two episodes of haemoptysis, and right-sided pleuritic chest pain. She
had been admitted 3 weeks earlier for treatment of exacerbation of COPD.

Past Medical History
Severe COPD
Osteoporosis

Social History
An 80-pack year smoking history—stopped smoking 6 months ago.
Lives with husband who works. Husband assists with activities of
   daily living. Daughter visits daily.
Exercise tolerance—SOB mobilising from room to room at home. Goes
   out in wheelchair.
Bathroom and bedroom downstairs.

Drug History
Salbutamol nebuliser
Tiotropium inhaler
Salmeterol inhaler
Alendronate
Vitamin D
Calcichew
   You are asked to review patient diagnosed with exacerbation of
COPD and hospital-acquired pneumonia. Respiratory function and
ABGs deteriorating. Productive of purulent sputum.

From the End of the Bed
Airway:
Spontaneous ventilation, airway patent. Speaking in short sentences.

Breathing:
Work of Breathing (WOB)
Respiratory pattern: paradoxical breathing, active expiration, accessory muscles active
RR 32 breaths per minute.
SpO_2 97% on 40% O_2 via face mask
Pleuritic pain on coughing

Circulation: BP 105/60 mmHg, HR 105 beats per minute, sinus rhythm, temperature 38.2° C.

Current Medical Management:
IV antibiotics
IV fluids
30mg prednisolone
Salbutamol and atrovent (ipratropium) nebulisers
40% O_2
Alendronate
Calcichew
Vitamin D

Investigations
Chest x-ray
Hyperinflated thorax, emphysematous bullae upper zones, shadowing and air bronchograms consistent with consolidation in right lower zone. Loss of medial half of right hemidiaphragm (silhouette sign).

Computed tomography of pulmonary artery (CTPA): Normal.

ABGs (on F_iO_2 0.4): pH 7.30, PaO_2 11.4 kPa, $PaCO_2$ 8.6 kPa, HCO_3^- 34 mmol/L, BE −4.4.

Bloods: haemoglobin (Hb) 165 g/L, white blood cell (WBC) 20 × 10^9/L, urea 12 mmol/L, creatinine 80 μmol/L.

Physical Examination
Palpation
Poor lower thoracic expansion (right >left) and upper thoracic movement consistent with hyperinflation.

Auscultation
Breath sounds (BS) quiet throughout with expiratory wheeze.
Further ↓BS, right lower zone.
Late inspiratory crackles, right lower zone.
Early expiratory crackles transmitting from upper airways.

Percussion note:
Dull right lower zone
Hyperresonant elsewhere.

Questions

1. What do you need to consider before treating this patient, based on assessment findings?
2. What are your treatment options?

Answers

1. The following factors need to be considered:

Type II respiratory failure
Is the O_2% appropriate? The high Hb is indicative of chronically low pO_2 (polycythaemia) and raised bicarbonate suggests chronically high $PaCO_2$ (chronic type II respiratory failure). This patient is likely to be oxygen sensitive and may have oxygen-induced respiratory acidosis. A target PaO_2 of 8 kPa is probably more realistic for this patient.

Pain
Ensure adequate analgesia before treatment.

Haemoptysis
When was the last episode of haemoptysis?
Were there streaks of blood (commonly associated with pneumonia) or was it frank haemoptysis? How will this affect your choice of treatment?
Note that pulmonary embolus has been ruled out by normal CTPA.
Is the patient being investigated for cancer of the lung?
You may want to check Hb levels.

Dehydration
The patient is dehydrated – raised urea with normal creatinine, low BP and HR. This will hinder sputum clearance.

Osteoporosis
Check CXR for fractures.
Care with manual techniques.

Emphysematous Bullae
There is an increased risk of pneumothorax with any positive pressure techniques in patients with bullous emphysema.

2. Treatment options:

Liaise with medical staff regarding O_2 therapy (see earlier). If patient is still in type II respiratory failure following controlled O_2 therapy to achieve a more realistic PaO_2, consider noninvasive ventilation (NIV). Note: there is a risk of pneumothorax with positive pressure treatments in patients with emphysematous bullae.

Humidify O_2, encourage oral fluids, consider saline nebulisers or mucolytics to assist with sputum clearance.

Increase emphasis on breathing control, in positions of ease, during active cycle of breathing techniques (ACBT).

If using manual techniques, reassess regularly to check that bronchospasm is not worsening, and use extra caution because of osteoporosis. Stop manual treatments if haemoptysis returns.

Use positioning to reduce WOB and optimise ventilation/perfusion (V/Q) matching. Modified positions may be required because of breathlessness.

CASE STUDY 4: SURGICAL WARD

History

A 62-year-old male with colon cancer, had an elective right hemicolectomy via a laparotomy incision 2 days ago. Seen by physiotherapist on first postoperative day when chest was noted to be clear, but he has become increasingly SOB at rest (SOBAR) since.

Past medical history

Normally fit and well.

Social History

Retired teacher, lives with wife, has two adult children; ex-smoker (30-pack year history, gave up 10 years ago), plays golf twice a week.

You have been asked to review as he is unable to expectorate, with an increasing respiratory rate suggestive of PPC.

From the End of the Bed

Airway

- SOBAR, able to speak short sentences.

Breathing

- RR 28, SpO2 94% on 8 L via simple low-flow face mask.

Circulation
- BP 162/85 mmHg, temperature 38.8° C, pulse 112 beats per minute.
- NBM (nil by mouth), IV fluid 100 mL/h.

Drug History
- Normally nil
- Since theatre:
  - Patient-controlled analgesia (PCA) morphine—not being used at regular intervals
  - Stemetil (prochlorperazine) IV—for nausea
  - Enoxaparin sodium subcutaneous injection—anticoagulant

Investigations
Electrocardiogram sinus tachycardia
ABGs: pH 7.39, PaO$_2$ 9.9, PaCO$_2$ 4.80, HCO$_3^-$ 23.1, BE –1.0
CXR: Poor inspiratory volume and likely R and L basal atelectasis
Blood counts: Hb 116, WCC 13.2.

Physical Examination
Palpation
Apical breathing, tactile fremitus over right middle zone anteriorly.

Auscultation
Quiet BS throughout especially at bases, few crackles in upper respiratory tract (URT).

Questions
1. What are the key assessment findings and why?
2. What are your treatment options?

Answers
1. Key assessment findings:

General
He was previously fit and well, but his past smoking history may have resulted in some residual mild COPD.

Cardiovascular System
HR and BP could suggest inadequate pain relief and/or infection. Increased WCC could indicate infection.

Respiratory

Poor lung expansion—suggesting atelectasis (CXR and auscultation)
Atelectasis and infection would produce falling oxygen saturations
Palpation and auscultation suggest some secretions
Oxygen is being delivered 'dry', this could contribute to the secretion retention and increase WOB

2. Treatment options:

Analgesia

Discuss with multidisciplinary team strategies to improve analgesia. Reassure him that you do not want to make the pain worse.

Respiratory

Discuss prescription and humidification with medical staff. Find admission saturation level, in view of possible COPD—you may have to accept a lower than normal value.
Consider saline nebulisers—consult with medical staff for prescription.
Position in high side lying to promote basal expansion.
Consider ACBT with wound support for coughing.

CASE STUDY 5: NEUROLOGIC UNIT

A 52-year-old man with progressive muscle weakness affecting all four limbs.
Past medical history
No previous hospital admissions, minor illnesses only.
Social history
Married, schoolteacher. Nonsmoker; usually very active.

Medical findings on admission
Alert, oriented
Cranial nerves—intact
Motor power—proximal muscle weakness grades 3 to 4
Sensation—intact

Respiratory System
Trachea central, respiratory rate 20 breaths per minute
Normal breath sounds
Vital capacity 5 L

CXR—elevated right hemidiaphragm
ABGs: pH 7.4, $PaCO_2$ 4.49, PaO_2 9.9 HCO_3- 22
   O_2 saturation 95% on air

Provisional Diagnosis

Guillain–Barré syndrome.
   Asked to see 6 hours after admission because vital capacity has fallen to 1.6 L; requiring 35% O_2 to maintain SpO_2 of 96%.

Questions

1. What further information will you require, and what will be the key elements of your assessment?
2. At this stage, what are your treatment options (management plan)?

Answers

1. Indications for physiotherapy:
   There has been a rapid and major deterioration in the patient's condition. Vital capacity has fallen by 68% from 5 to 1.6 L. The patient's ability to take a sigh breath is impaired, as is their ability to clear any retained secretions. Some degree of atelectasis will have already occurred. This will probably progress to major lobar collapse and sputum retention.
   At admission, there were already signs that would have predicted the possibility of respiratory deterioration:
   1.1 The elevated right diaphragm in the absence of obvious lobar collapse suggests that there is some degree of paralysis of this muscle.
   1.2 The high respiratory rate and low CO_2 suggest that the patient is working very hard to maintain his PaO_2 and oxygen saturation levels at 96%.
   Without intervention, this patient is likely to fatigue quickly and progress to respiratory failure and require ventilation.
2. Further information required:
   Observe and assess the patient.
   ABGs are essential; the patient may already be retaining CO_2.
   Repeat CXR.
   Is there any indication that the patient may be at risk of aspiration, for example, wet-sounding voice, reports of coughing when drinking?
3. Treatment options:
   Position the patient so as to reduce the WOB (see Chapter 7).

Humidify oxygen.

Reassure the patient.

Intermittent positive pressure breathing (IPPB) to inflate lung and improve lung compliance thus reducing the work of breathing and oxygen demand.

Patient review in 1 hour; repeat vital capacity and ABGs.

If CO_2 continues to rise, ventilation will need to be discussed. Depending on the team decision this may be NIV, if available, or full ventilation. Care must be taken not to mask a deteriorating patient—close monitoring is essential.

May benefit from cough augmentation, manual assisted cough or cough assist

Review as planned.

Inform staff of current action plan and leave contact number.

If patient's condition stabilises or improves, continue with current treatment plan and monitoring.

Ensure the ICU has been alerted to the problem. If the patient continues to deteriorate, a planned intubation is preferable to an emergency intubation.

CASE STUDY 6: CARDIOTHORACIC WARD

A 69-year-old man, postcoronary artery bypass grafting yesterday. Initially well and mobilised to chair this morning; however, during this evening he has become more breathless, hypoxic and anxious. He has never smoked.

You are called in to see him and when you arrive

He has a PCA morphine but is anxious, tense and complaining of pain

Obese gentleman, slumped in bed

BP 100/60 mmHg, HR 110 sinus tachycardia (ST), central venous pressure 12

Bloods—WCC 14.5, Hb 100 g/L, c-reactive protein (CRP) 150, albumin 24

UO 20 mL per hour, last 3 hours. Fluid balance positive 2 L

- Self-ventilating on 98% O_2 via face mask (humidified), RR 25 (laboured), SpO_2 92%.
- Auscultation: barely audible breath sounds basally with a few late inspiratory crackles. Equal but poor chest expansion

ABGs—pH 7.37, PaO_2 8.2 kPa, $PaCO_2$ 4.5 kPa, HCO_3^- 22, BE +1

CXR—awaited.

Questions

1. What are his main physio problems?
2. What are his main medical problems?
3. What might prevent you from mobilising this patient?
4. What can you do?
5. What would you like to discuss with his doctors?
6. What objective markers could you use to assess change?

Answers

1. Pain, bilateral basal collapse, increased work of breathing, reduced expansion, anxiety, hypoxia
2. Inadequate pain control, hypotension (likely causing poor renal function), pulmonary oedema, potential infection brewing
3. Minimal respiratory reserve, pain and anxiety (see Chapter 7 Work of breathing), hypotension (likely to worsen when upright)
4. Reassure and reposition; if upright sitting, ensure abdomen does not impinge on diaphragmatic excursion. Continuous positive airway pressure (CPAP) —check CXR first. Remember his size: he will need big PEEP (10 cmH$_2$O) and a high flow to meet his inspiratory flow demand. Will also need a high O$_2$ until an improvement in ABGs is evident
5. Optimisation of analgesia and review of poor urine output. Discuss use of CPAP and possible movement to a higher level of care
6. Auscultation, ABGs, O$_2$%, SpO$_2$, RR and WOB

CASE STUDY 7: THORACIC UNIT

A 45-year-old woman had a left lower lobectomy 2 days ago. She has good pain control using an epidural but is unable to clear sputum. She gave up heavy smoking 8 weeks ago.

On Arrival

- Patient sat in chair.
- BP 110/75 mmHg, HR 80 SR, adequate urine output, fluid balance positive 500 mL.
- Spontaneous breathing on 4 L O$_2$ via nasal canulae, SpO$_2$ 94%, RR 18 normal pattern, cough wet and weak. Palpable fremitus on anterior chest wall and poor expansion on left. Auscultation: widespread transmitted coarse expiratory crackles, with reduced breath sounds left lower zone. Two chest drains in situ (one api-

cal, one basal). Apical chest drain is bubbling —both drains are on suction.

Questions
1. Why is the apical chest drain bubbling?
2. What are her physio problems?
3. What are your treatment options?

Answers
1. Failure of the pleura to stick up postoperatively because of a persistent air leak from the lung into the intrapleural space.
2. Secretion retention, poor tidal volume.
3. Mobilise (check chest drains can come off suction) – to increase her tidal volumes. If she is on strict suction, march on spot, or use exercise bike (if possible). Supported coughing/huffing to aid sputum clearance. Consider nebulisers (saline or salbutamol) for really sticky sputum and consider changing to humidified oxygen therapy.

CASE STUDY 8: HAEMATOLOGY WARD

Background
A 75-year-old male, with a long history of chronic lymphocytic leukaemia (CLL), had donor bone marrow transplant 3 months ago. Admitted yesterday unwell with a 3- to 4-day history of persistent dry cough and SOB on exertion. Asked to review as deteriorating respiratory symptoms with CXR changes. Doctors asked for sputum specimen.

Past Medical History
Ten years ago, CLL—had an autograft (own bone marrow transplant) with chemotherapy and total body irradiation (TBI).

Social History
Lives with wife, two adult children, lifelong nonsmoker.

On arrival
A—SOBAR, unable to speak full sentences
B—RR 32, SpO$_2$ 92% on O$_2$ 60% via face mask

C—BP 95/60 mmHg; temperature 38.5º C; pulse 126 beats per minute (ST)
   Fluids in progress.

Drug History
Immunosuppressants.

Investigations
ABGs: pH 7.24, pCO_2 4.80, PO_2 11.4, HCO_3^- 14.9, BE −11.0
CXR shows bilateral basal consolidation
Blood counts: Hb 9.3, WCC 0.2, platelets 22.

Auscultation/palpation
Harsh BS throughout with bilateral basal crackles
Apical expansion only.

Questions
1. What are the key findings of your assessment and why?
2. What are your treatment options?

Answers
1. Key assessment findings:

General
Because of long treatment history, consider fatigue and nutritional
status.

Cardiovascular system
Note tachycardia with a low BP and pyrexia. This patient is exhibit-
ing signs of sepsis (be aware, immunosuppressants may mask signs of
infection as they keep WCC low).
   Review blood counts and be aware of the implications of low platelets.
A low WCC may result in low sputum production (atypical infection).

Respiratory
Previous radiotherapy may cause fibrotic changes to lungs.
ABGs: is patient compensating for a metabolic acidosis with an
   increased respiratory rate?
2. Treatment options:
   Recognise extreme limitations because of cardiovascular instability.

You could position to reduce WOB, and CPAP may be appropriate. However, this patient needs senior medical review and potentially more invasive support.

CASE STUDY 9: ONCOLOGY WARD

A 73-year-old woman with squamous cell carcinoma (SCC) of oesophagus. Three weeks postoesophageal bypass procedure with a feeding jejunostomy for radiotherapy-induced oesophageal stricture. Postoperative recovery complicated by left vocal cord palsy. It is thought she has aspirated, causing respiratory distress. Although the speech and language therapist recommended NBM, specialist registrar deemed patient safe for soft diet.

Past Medical History
SCC oesophagus diagnosed 6 years previously, treated with chemotherapy and radiotherapy.
Breast cancer 25 years ago, known single pulmonary metastasis.

Social History
Widow, lives with son. Ex-smoker.

On Arrival
A—SOB, 'wet' incoherent voice
B—RR 22, SpO$_2$ 84% on humidified O$_2$ 90% via face mask
C—BP 151/70 mmHg; temperature 36.3° C; pulse 102 beats per minute (ST).

Drug History
Tamoxifen.

Investigations
ABGs: pH 7.42, PaO$_2$ 8.32, PaCO$_2$ 6.38, HCO$_3^-$ 29.8, BE +6.5
CXR shows right middle lobe patchy shadowing
Blood counts: Hb 95, WCC 17.0, platelets 185, CRP 284.

Auscultation/Palpation
Widespread coarse crackles with tactile fremitus.

Questions

1. What are the key assessment findings and why?
2. What are your treatment options?

Answers

1. Key assessment findings:

General

Sudden deterioration

Recent oesophageal surgery—note altered anatomy and contraindica-
tions/cautions to treatment

Long history of swallowing difficulties.

Cardiovascular System

Signs of infection – tachycardia with raised WCC and CRP.

Central Nervous System

Signs of confusion, could be caused by:

hypoxia

neurological event

brain metastases

Respiratory

Single pulmonary metastasis (be aware of)

2. Treatment options:

  Ascertain if appropriate for critical care and resus status. She is
  acutely unwell and needs immediate action to avoid further
  deterioration.

  Liaise with medical team regarding suction and IPPB. Needs to
  be documented before undertaking these treatments because of
  altered anatomy and risk of damage to anastomosis.

  May be too fatigued and confused for ACBT and has an ineffective
  cough because of vocal cord palsy. Therefore positioning, manual
  techniques and suction (if team consent) may be only options.

CASE STUDY 10: PAEDIATRIC WARD

An 18-month-old child admitted to ward with chest infection.

History of present condition: Admitted today with 1/7 history of irritability, cough, increased WOB, pyrexia.

Past medical history
Suspected gastro-oesophageal reflux.
Drug history: cefuroxime, omeprazole, paracetamol, 0.9% saline nebs
Observation Supine

  RR—30 breaths per minute
  SpO_2—90%
  O_2 —5 L, dry, O_2 via mask
  HR—157 beats per minute
  BP—105/69 mmHg
  CRT—1 second
  Temperature—38.0º C
  Increased WOB (subcostal recession, nasal flare)
  Symmetrical expansion, nil palpable
  Auscultation—Bronchial breath sounds throughout right lung
  Cap gas pH 7.34, PaO_2 6 kPa, $PaCO_2$ 6.7 kPa, HCO_3 26.7, BE +2.5
  CXR—Taken today (see Fig, 19.1)
  Weight – 8 kg
  Alert and responsive
  CXR (taken today)

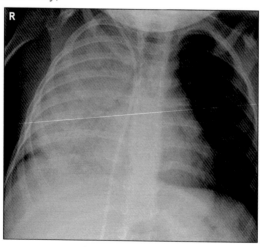

Questions

1. What are the abnormal markers?
2. What does auscultation suggest?
3. What does CXR show?
4. Interpret blood gas. What does it show?

5. Are there any cautions/contraindications?
6. What interventions would you perform?
7. What other intervention or advice would you give?

Answers

1. Respiratory distress (tachypnoea, recession, nasal flare, low saturations), tachycardia and auscultation changes. Patient unwell and likely to tire further unless appropriate intervention received.
2. Acute consolidation right lung
3. Consolidated right lung (air bronchograms, no volume loss)
4. Type 2 respiratory failure.
5. Manual chest physiotherapy may increase inflammation therefore is not indicated. Avoid left side lying, may increase WOB
6. Improve oxygenation. Commence heated high flow humidified oxygen at an appropriate flow for the patient's weight and titrate the oxygen, according to saturations (Start at 16 L flow and 70% O_2)
7. Change position to prone—maximise ventilation/perfusion matching (close monitoring)

   Consider right side lying—maximise ventilation to the left lung.

   If URT secretions palpable/audible—consider effectiveness of cough

   If cough is weak—consider nasopharyngeal suction

   Advise nursing staff—reposition regularly between prone and right side lying and nasopharyngeal suction if required.

USEFUL ABBREVIATIONS

A&E: Accident & Emergency
ABCDE: Airway, Breathing, Circulation, Disability, Exposure
ABG: arterial blood gas
ACBT: active cycle of breathing techniques
ACE: angiotensin converting enzyme
ACPRC: Association of Chartered Physiotherapists in Respiratory Care
ACT: airway clearance technique
AD: autogenic drainage
AF: atrial fibrillation
ALI: acute lung injury
AML: acute myeloid leukaemia
AP: anteroposterior
APTT: activated partial thromboplastin time
APRV: airway pressure release ventilation
ARDS: acute respiratory distress syndrome
ASAP: as soon as possible
ASB: assisted spontaneous breathing
ASD: atrial septal defect
ASIA: American spinal injury association
Ausc.: auscultation
AV: atrioventricular
ACVPU: Alert, Confused, responding to Voice, Pain or is Unresponsive
AVSD: atrioventricular septal defect
AVR: aortic valve replacement
BAL: bronchoalveolar lavage
BC: breathing control
BE: base excess
BiPAP: bi-level positive airway pressure
BLS: basic life support
BMI: body mass index
BOS: base of skull
BP: blood pressure (arterial)

BPD: bronchopulmonary dysplasia
BS: breath sounds
BTS: British Thoracic Society
Ca: cancer
CABG: coronary artery bypass graft
CAL: chronic airflow limitation
CAP: community acquired pneumonia
CCF: congestive cardiac failure
CF: cystic fibrosis
CFM: cerebral function monitor
CHD: congenital heart disease
CHD: coronary heart disease
CHF: chronic heart failure
CMD: congenital muscular dystrophy
CMV: continuous mandatory ventilation
CMV: cytomegalovirus
CNS: central nervous system
CO: cardiac output
CO_2: carbon dioxide
COAD: chronic obstructive airway disease
COPD: chronic obstructive pulmonary disease
CP: cerebral palsy
CPD: continuing professional development
CPAP: continuous positive airway pressure
CPAx: Chelsea Critical Care Physiotherapy Assessment Tool
CPP: cerebral perfusion pressure
CRP: C-reactive protein
CRT: capillary refill time
CSF: cerebrospinal fluid
CSP: Chartered Society of Physiotherapy
CT: computed tomography
CVA: cerebrovascular accident
CVVHD: continuous veno-venous haemodialysis
CVVHF: continuous veno-venous haemofiltration
CVP: central venous pressure
CVS: cardiovascular system
CXR: chest x-ray
DBE: deep breathing exercises
DH: drug history
DIC: disseminated intravascular coagulation

DKA: diabetic ketoacidosis
DMD: Duchenne muscular dystrophy
DVT: deep vein thrombosis
ECG: electrocardiogram
ECMO: extracorporeal membrane oxygenation
EGDT: early goal directed therapy
ENT: ear, nose & throat
EMG: electromyography
EPAP: expiratory positive airway pressure
ERAS: enhanced recovery after surgery
ET: endotracheal
ETT: endotracheal tube
EVAR: endovascular aneurysm repair
EVD: external ventricular drain
EWS: early warning score
FBC: full blood count
Fen.: fenestrated
FET: forced expiration technique
FEV_1: forced vital capacity in first second of expiration
FH: family history
FiO_2: fraction of inspired oxygen
FRC: functional residual capacity
FVC: forced vital capacity
GA: general anaesthetic
GAP: gravity-assisted positioning
GCS: Glasgow Coma Scale
GI: gastrointestinal
GOR: gastrooesophageal reflux
GTN: glyceryl trinitrate
Hb: haemoglobin
HCO_3^-: bicarbonate
HDU: high dependency unit
HF: haemofiltration
HFNC: high flow nasal cannula
HFO: high-frequency oscillation
HFOV: high-frequency oscillatory ventilation
HME: heat and moisture exchanger
HPC: history of present condition
HR: heart rate
HRCT: high resolution computerized tomography

IABP: intraaortic balloon pump
ICD: intercostal drain
ICP: intracranial pressure
ICU: intensive care unit
ICU-AW: intensive care unit—acquired weakness
IHD: ischaemic heart disease
ILD: Interstitial lung disease
IM: intramuscular
IMT: inspiratory muscle training
INR: international normalized ratio
IPAP: inspiratory positive airway pressure
IPPB: intermittent positive pressure breathing
IPPV: intermittent positive pressure ventilation
IS: incentive spirometry
IV: intravenous
JVP: jugular venous pressure
K$^+$: potassium ions
LFT: lung function test *or* liver function test
LLL: left lower lobe
LOS: length of stay
LPA: lasting power of attorney
LRTI: lower respiratory tract infection
LTEE: lower thoracic expansion exercise
LTOT: long-term oxygen therapy
LUL: left upper lobe
LVAD: left ventricular assist device
LVF: left ventricular failure
LZ: lower zone
MAP: mean arterial pressure
MDT: multidisciplinary team
MHI: manual hyperinflation
MI: myocardial infarction
MIP: maximal inspiratory pressure
MR: mitral regurgitation
MRI: magnetic resonance imaging
MRSA: methicillin-resistant *Staphylococcus aureus*
MT: manual techniques
MV: minute volume
MVR: mitral valve replacement
MZ: middle zone

Na^+: sodium ions
NaCl: sodium chloride
NAI: nonaccidental injury
NBM: nil by mouth
NCA: nurse-controlled analgesia
NGT: nasogastric tube
NIBP: noninvasive blood pressure
NICU: neonatal intensive care unit
NIPPV: noninvasive intermittent positive pressure ventilation
NIV: noninvasive ventilation
NJ: nasojejunostomy
NO: nitric oxide
NP: nasopharyngeal
NSAIDs: nonsteroidal antiinflammatory drugs
NSTEMI: non ST segment elevation myocardial infarction
O_2: oxygen
OP: oropharyngeal
OPCAB: off pump coronary artery bypass
OSA: obstructive sleep apnoea
PA: pulmonary artery
PA: posteroanterior
$PaCO_2$: partial pressure of carbon dioxide in arterial blood
PACS: picture archiving and communication systems
PaO_2: partial pressure of oxygen in arterial blood
PAP: peak airway pressure
PAWP: pulmonary artery wedge pressure
PCA: patient-controlled analgesia
PCD: primary ciliary dyskinesia
PCEA: patient-controlled epidural anaesthesia/analgesia
PCF: peak cough flow
PCI: percutaneous coronary intervention
PCP: *Pneumocystis carinii* pneumonia
PCPAP: periodic CPAP
PD: postural drainage
PDP: personal development plan
PE: pulmonary embolus
PEEP: positive end expiratory pressure
PEFR: peak expiratory flow rate
PEG: percutaneous endoscopic gastrostomy
PEP: positive expiratory pressure

PERL/PEARL: pupils equal and reactive to light
PET: positron emission tomography
pH: negative logarithm of hydrogen ion concentration in moles per litre
PICC: peripherally inserted central catheter
PICU: paediatric intensive care unit
PIP: positive inspiratory pressure
Plts: platelets
PMH: past medical history
PND: paroxysmal nocturnal dyspnoea
PPC: postoperative pulmonary complications
PPM: permanent pacemaker
PRN: 'as required'
PRVC: pressure-regulated volume control
PS: pressure support *or* pulmonary stenosis
PT: prothrombin time
PVC: premature ventricular contraction
PVD: peripheral vascular disease
QOL: quality of life
RBC: red blood count
RLL: right lower lobe
RML: right middle lobe
RPE: rating of perceived exertion
RR: respiratory rate
RS: respiratory system
RSV: respiratory syncytial virus
RTA: road traffic accident
RUL: right upper lobe
SA: sinoatrial
SABA: short acting beta agonist
SAH: subarachnoid haemorrhage
SaO_2: saturation of oxygen in arterial blood (shown in ABGs)
SB: spina bifida
SBOT: short burst oxygen therapy
SBP: systolic blood pressure
SC: subcutaneous
SCI: spinal cord injury
SH: social history
SIMV: synchronized mandatory ventilation
SIRS: systemic inflammatory response syndrome
SMA: spinal muscular atrophy

SOB: shortness of breath
SOBAR: shortness of breath at rest
SOBOE: shortness of breath on exertion
SpO_2: pulse oximetry arterial oxygen saturation
SR: sinus rhythm
SSC: squamous cell carcinoma
ST: sinus tachycardia
STEMI: ST-segment elevation myocardial infarction
STOT: short-term oxygen therapy
SV: self-ventilating/stroke volume
SVCO: superior vena cava obstruction
TAVI: transcatheter aortic valve implantation
TB: tuberculosis
TBI: traumatic brain injury/total body irradiation
TEE: thoracic expansion exercise
TENS: transcutaneous electrical nerve stimulation
TGA: transposition of great arteries
TMR: transmyocardial revascularization
TOE: transoesophageal echocardiogram
TOF: tetralogy of Fallot
TPN: total parental nutrition
TV: tidal volume
UAS: upper abdominal surgery
UO: urinary output
URT: upper respiratory tract
UWSD: underwater sealed drainage
UZ: upper zone
V_T: tidal volume
VAD: ventricular assist device
VAP: ventilator associated pneumonia
VAS: visual analogue scale
VATS: video assisted thoracic surgery
VC: vital capacity
VHI: ventilator hyperinflation
VILI: ventilator induced lung injury
V/Q: ventilation/perfusion ratio
VSD: ventricular septal defect
VTE: venous thromboembolism
WCC: white cell count
WOB: work of breathing

NORMAL VALUES

There are variations in published normal values. The ranges quoted in your hospital/facility/trust should be used in practice.

AGE GROUP	HEART RATE— MEAN (RANGE) BEATS PER MINUTE	RESPIRATORY RATE—RANGE BREATHS PER MINUTE	BLOOD PRESSURE— SYSTOLIC/ DIASTOLIC (MMHG)
Preterm	150 (100–200)	40–60	39–59/16–36
Newborn	140 (80–200)	30–50	50–70/25–45
<2 years	130 (100–190)	20–40	87–105/53–66
>2 years	80 (60–140)	20–40	95–105/53–66
>6 years	75 (60–90)	15–30	97–112/57–71
Adult	70 (50–100)	12–16	95–140/60–90

Normal value of mean arterial pressure
Diastolic + [(Systolic − Diastolic)/3] = 70–110 mmHg

Normal values for central venous pressure (CVP) and intracranial pressure (ICP)
Normal CVP: 3–8 mmHg
Normal ICP: <10 mmHg

From Main and Denhey (2016) Cardiorespiratory Physiotherapy 5th edition London Elsevier

Blood Gases

	NEWBORN	UP TO 3 YEARS	3–6 YEARS	>6 YEARS	ADULT
Arterial blood pH	7.30–7.40	7.30–7.40	7.35–7.45	7.35–7.45	7.35–7.45
$PaCO_2$ mmHg kPa	30–35 4.0–4.7	30–35 4.0–4.7	35–45 4.7–6.0	35–45 4.7–6.0	35–45 4.7–6.0
PaO_2 mmHg kPa	60–90 8.0–12.0	80–100 10.7–13.3	80–100 10.7–13.3	80–100 10.7–13.3	80–100 10.7–13.3
$HCO3^-$ mmol/L	22–26	22–26	22–26	22–26	22–26
Base excess	−2 to +2	−2 to +2	−2 to +2	−2 to +2	−2 to +2

Normal values for venous blood
   PH 7.31–7.41 [H+] 46–38 nmol/L
   PO_2 5.0–5.6 kPa (37–42 mmHg)
   PCO_2 5.6–6.7 kPa (42–50 mmHg)

From: Main and Denhey (2016) Cardiorespiratory Physiotherapy 5th Edition London. Elsevier

CONVERSION TABLES

0.133 KPA = 51. MMHG		PH = 9- LOG [H+] WHERE [H+] IS IN NMOL/L	
KPA	MMHG	PH	[H+]
1	7.5	7.52	30
2	15.0	7.45	35
4	30	7.40	40
6	45	7.35	45
8	60	7.30	50
10	75	7.26	55
12	90	7.22	60
14	105	7.19	65

From Main and Denhey Cardiorespiratory Physiotherapy 5th edition London Elsevier

Blood chemistry

Albumin	37–53 g/L
Calcium (Ca^{2+})	2.25–2.65 mmol/L
Creatinine	60–120 mmol/L
Glucose	4–6 mmol/L
Potassium (K$^+$)	3.4–5.0 mmol/L
Sodium (Na$^+$)	134–140 mmol/L
Urea	2.5–6.5 mmol/L
Haemoglobin (Hb)	14.0–18.0 g/100 mL (men)
	11.5–15.5 g/100 mL (women)
Platelets	150–400 × 10^9/L
White blood cell count (WCC)	4–11 10^9/L
Urine output	1 mL/kg/h

From: Main and Denhey (2016) Cardiorespiratory Physiotherapy 5th edition London Elsevier

SURGICAL INCISIONS

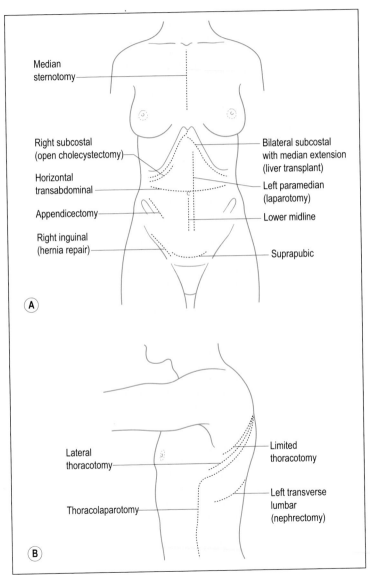

Fig. A.1 ● Figure showing common surgical incisions.
Reproduced from Pryor and Prasad (2002), with kind permission.
NOTE! With certain surgeries patients may have more than one surgical incision!

Note: Page numbers followed by "f" indicate figures "t" indicate tables and "b" indicate boxes.